Schizophrenia and Genetics

Schizophrenia is a widely investigated psychiatric condition, and though there have been claims of gene "associations," decades of molecular genetic studies have failed to produce confirmed causative genes. In this book, Joseph focuses on the methodological shortcomings of schizophrenia genetic research.

His findings have major implications not only on how we understand the causes of schizophrenia and other psychaitric conditions, but also on how we understand the causes of human behavior in general. Chapters explore the differing theoretical concepts of schizophrenia, molecular genetic research around schizophrenia, family, twin, and adoption studies, and non-medical prevention and intervention strategies. Prominent researchers and studies in the field are discussed and critiqued comprehensively throughout.

This book is essential reading for psychiatrists, psychologists, behavioral scientists, and anyone interested in the causes of human behavior.

Jay Joseph, Psy.D. is a clinical psychologist practicing in the San Francisco Bay Area. He is the author of three previous books, most recently *The Trouble with Twin Studies: A Reassessment of Twin Research in the Social and Behavioral Sciences.*

Schizophrenia and Genetics
The End of An Illusion

Jay Joseph

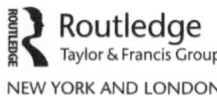
Routledge
Taylor & Francis Group

NEW YORK AND LONDON

First Spanish edition published by Herder 2021
First English edition published by Routledge 2023

ISBN: 978-1-032-27552-9 (hbk)
ISBN: 978-1-032-27550-5 (pbk)
ISBN: 978-1-003-29327-9 (ebk)

DOI: 10.4324/9781003293279

Typeset in Sabon
by Deanta Global Publishing Services, Chennai, India

Contents

Tables

Figures

Preface

I became interested in the "genetics of schizophrenia" topic as a clinical psychology graduate student in the mid-1990s. The arguments fascinated me, and because I saw the genetic argument as weak, it was stunning to hear that the debate had been largely closed in favor of genetics by the 1980s. How is that possible, I asked myself. I decided to focus my 1998 doctoral dissertation on a critical analysis of schizophrenia genetic research. At that time, it seemed obvious to me that twin studies proved nothing about genetic influences on behavior, yet every textbook I picked up said that twin studies provided conclusive evidence in favor of genetics. Something wasn't right. I wanted to learn more about genetic research, which led me to the writings of critics of the mental health system and the medical model of human distress and dysfunction. I discovered several authors who had written critically about genetic research in psychiatry and psychology, and their work inspired me to look more closely at the original studies, including the adoption studies I review in Chapter 6. Aided by what previous critics had said about them, when I read these adoption studies closely, I was amazed to discover that they too were cited favorably in most textbooks.

I have been writing critically about behavioral twin studies, in both their reared-together and "reared-apart" forms, since the late 1990s, including a book I published with Routledge on that topic in 2015, *The Trouble with Twin Studies: A Reassessment of Twin Research in the Social and Behavioral Sciences*. Since 1998 I have published other books, chapters, online articles, and peer-reviewed academic journal articles on genetic research and theories in the social and behavioral sciences. Apart from my unpublished dissertation, this is my first book focused entirely on schizophrenia. A major theme of my work has been that if we put behavioral genetic and psychiatric genetic research under the microscope, the main findings and theories produced by these fields do not hold up. Although some themes and topics from my earlier books are also found in this book, here I present an up-to-date and revised analysis integrating concepts and terms developed in the "replication crisis" in science, where research publications, including famous ones, have come under increasing scrutiny. Schizophrenia genetic research can now be assessed and deconstructed using replication crisis terms and concepts.

I am a clinical psychologist practicing in the San Francisco Bay Area of California. You could say that I do my critical genetics work "on the side," assisted by a few amazing supportive colleagues. Like other psychotherapists, in my clinical work I see harm done to people by their environments all the time. I have yet to work with people or families that have been directly harmed by supposed "genes for mental illness," but some have been harmed by being told they carry such genes.

In this book, I describe the main topics and controversies in ways that can be understood by people with a basic understanding of how science works and with some understanding of psychiatric diagnoses and concepts. I am confident that readers will find my analysis refreshingly original compared with the predicable, and usually uncritical academic and journalistic accounts of schizophrenia genetic research. Due to significant revisions, the text differs considerably from the 2021 Spanish language edition.

In the chapters that follow, I will show that the evidence psychiatry ceaselessly puts forward in support of schizophrenia as a genetic disorder is stunningly weak, a conclusion that has major implications for prevention and intervention strategies. This conclusion also has major implications for other areas of psychiatry and human behavior, and bears directly on the larger "nature-nurture" question. Science is about data, but more importantly about how scientists and others *interpret* data and the stories they tell about it. In this book, I tell a very different story from the one that students and the public are usually told, with the hope of helping inspire new generations of critical thinkers in the area of genetics and human behavior.

Jay Joseph, Psy.D.
Oakland, California, USA
September 2022

Acknowledgments

I dedicate this book to the memory of my late colleagues Steve Baldwin, David H. Jacobs, and Loren Mosher, who worked tirelessly to challenge medical model approaches to human behavior. Several people provided important assistance while I was writing this book. In particular, I want to thank Mike Jones, who was a student of family systems pioneer Murray Bowen and later a front-line general psychiatrist in community mental health, for providing valuable and insightful feedback. Mike read and commented on each chapter and helped make each one better. This is especially true for Chapter 2, given Mike's extensive knowledge of psychiatric molecular genetic research. He also offered keen insights in relation to the *Hidden Valley Road* and *Genain Quadruplets* stories found in Chapters 3 and 5, respectively. Mary Boyle also provided valuable feedback and assistance on two key chapters.

Several other colleagues read chapters and provided additional valuable feedback. These colleagues include David Cohen, Duncan Double, Roar Fosse, Jonathan Leo, Steve Pittelli, and Ken Richardson. Correspondence with Victor Lidz, Charles Lidz, and Jerry Lidz helped me better understand the atmosphere of 1970s and 1980s American psychiatry. I would also like to thank Robert Whitaker, creator of the *Mad in America* website, for providing space for me to publish online articles on that site since 2013. I thank Taylor and Francis Mental Health Editor Sarah Gore for helping make this book possible, and Mental Health Editorial Assistant Upasruti Biswas for help in the early stages. I thank my family for their patience and understanding as I was working on this book.

I should be clear that all conclusions I reach and opinions I express in this book are entirely my own, and do not necessarily reflect the views of people who helped along the way. In addition, any errors are entirely my responsibility. Unless otherwise noted, all italicized words and phrases appearing in quotations are those of the quoted authors.

1 Introduction

In a 2003 edition of *Science*, one of the world's leading scientific journals, the editors declared that the identification of "mental illness" genes was the second most important "scientific breakthrough" of the year. "Schizophrenia, depression, and bipolar disorder often run in families," the editors wrote, "but only recently have researchers identified particular genes that reliably increase one's risk of disease." The prefrontal cortex, they wrote, "is regulated in part by a gene called COMT, one of the handful associated with risk of schizophrenia."[1] As it turned out, claims based on these "particular genes" didn't hold up, including the COMT gene.[2] If a journal as prestigious as *Science* says that genes for psychiatric conditions have been discovered, most people take this as fact—and remember it as fact. But in this case, it turned out not to be a fact.

In both the popular and scientific literature, and in this book, the word "gene" (as in "genes for height" or "genes for IQ") is used as a shorthand for any form of DNA sequence variation that is associated with variation in some human characteristic. In this book I use the "gene" shorthand to describe genetic variation that is associated with the behavioral syndrome known as schizophrenia.

Despite the development of new methodologies leading to claims of gene associations based on the "genome-wide association" (GWAS) and "polygenic risk score" (PRS) studies I will explore in Chapter 2, genes shown to cause schizophrenia remain undiscovered. Nevertheless, mainstream authors believe that the evidence produced by family, twin, and adoption studies converges on the "high heritability" genetic basis of schizophrenia and psychosis, providing justification for continuing gene searches at the molecular genetic level. For mainstream researchers and commentators, the evidence seems so overwhelming that it is hard to imagine that anyone could suggest otherwise. In this book, I do suggest otherwise, and I will explore the "genetics of schizophrenia" literature from a totally different perspective from that found in most academic and journalistic accounts.

But why would someone want to read an entire book focused on the genetics of schizophrenia debate, a debate that most people think was settled in favor of genetics decades ago? One answer is that although I focus

DOI: 10.4324/9781003293279-1

on schizophrenia genetic research, the critique applies to other areas of psychiatry because similar methods are used across different diagnostic categories. As professor of anatomy Jonathan Leo, a critic of biological psychiatry, wrote in 2016, "Schizophrenia holds a unique spot in the annals of mental health research because of its perceived anatomical underpinnings, and is often cited as evidence in favor of a genetic predisposition to other conditions."[3]

More importantly, the "genetics of schizophrenia" question bears directly on the much wider long-running "nature-nurture" debate—a debate focused on the question of whether hereditary or environmental influences are the main cause of differences in human behavior and ability. In addition to other psychiatric conditions, the methods and concepts I examine in this book are used to support claims of important genetic influences in areas such as IQ, personality, criminal behavior, and all other areas of studied human behavior. Twin studies supposedly supply the main genetic evidence in these areas, and I explore the disputed key assumption of twin research in Chapters 4 and 5. The aim of this book, then, extends far beyond schizophrenia and psychiatry and into the larger question of what makes us human and whether our fates are largely determined by the genes we inherit.

If the mainstream "genetics of schizophrenia" story is wrong, the question then becomes why so many people still believe it. I will show in the chapters to come that this story—as well as the mainstream story of the genetics of most other areas of human behavior—follows a seven-step process. Twenty-five years of study has led me to conclude that this is a corrupted process, and it goes something like this: academic researchers in the fields of behavioral genetics and psychiatric genetics produce unsound research based on false assumptions and/or manipulated or genetically misinterpreted data, which is then accepted for publication in peer-reviewed academic journals → researchers producing this unsound research are rewarded, funded, tenured, and even honored, which motivates them to produce even more unsound research, sometimes over an entire career → respected academic fields endorse and promote this unsound research in textbooks and other publications → the mainstream (corporate) media reports on and promotes this unsound research, often in the form of articles and news reports of new discoveries based mainly on twin research → the mainstream media regularly reports on supposedly exciting new molecular genetic behavioral gene discoveries as if decades of non-replicated false-alarm claims had never happened → books written by journalists and some highly respected researchers and authors promote and celebrate unsound research → students and teachers in the academic world, political policy makers, and the general public are convinced by the above process that what are in fact unsound studies and false-alarm or non-causative behavioral gene discovery claims are actually sound studies and true causative gene discoveries. This leads them to accept and possibly promote various related political, social policy, scientific, and social-relations viewpoints.

If, instead, the "schizophrenia as a highly heritable disease" story is untrue, this could lead to the unraveling of claims that heredity plays a major role in determining human behavioral differences in general, an unraveling that surely would constitute a pivotal development in the history of the behavioral sciences. Society and science could then focus attention on *non*-genetic determinants of behavior, including those related to family, social, cultural, political, and economic environments, which would include an examination of how oppressive aspects of society cause psychological harm. This is one aspect of the "Power Threat Meaning Framework" (PTMF), which I will briefly discuss in the final chapter.[4]

This book will closely examine one important slice of a larger story of how the economically and politically powerful, as well as drug companies selling highly profitable psychiatric drugs, use genetic theories to sell us stories that help maintain a social, economic, and political status quo that benefits them and harms most of the rest of us. Although a detailed analysis of studies, theories, assumptions, and concepts is unavoidable, I will do my best to tell the story as clearly and interestingly as possible, including analyses of families affected by psychosis, and famous authors who are stunningly unfamiliar with the genetic studies they champion in their books. I will explore a tragic story of extreme abuse that led a set of identical quadruplets to all be diagnosed with schizophrenia in their early adult life. A famous American filmmaker will even make an appearance. In the final chapter I will examine alternative understandings of, and approaches to, schizophrenia and psychosis.

Before heading into these areas, in the remaining part of this chapter I will explore differing conceptions of schizophrenia, describe the field of psychiatric genetics, review evidence in support of environmental causes, describe some problems with genetic explanations of schizophrenia, and briefly review claims that schizophrenia is a brain disease. Finally, I will describe the questionable research practices that brought about the ongoing "replication crisis" in science. I will show in later chapters how these practices were sometimes used in schizophrenia genetic research.

Differing Conceptions of "Schizophrenia"

Kraepelin and Bleuler

The schizophrenia story begins with the creation of a medical disorder lacking evidence of a medical disease process. The diagnosis/term *dementia praecox* (dementia of early life) was developed by the German psychiatrist Emil Kraepelin (1856–1926) in the late 19th century. Kraepelin created dementia praecox by combining three existing categories into one, which he viewed as a progressively deteriorating brain disease.[5] These three conditions were called "hebephrenia," "vesania typica," and "catatonia." Kraepelin saw dementia praecox as a disease that eventually led to dementia.[6]

In 1911, the Swiss psychiatrist Eugen Bleuler (1857–1939) published *Dementia Praecox or the Group of Schizophrenias.* He coined the term *schizophrenia*, meaning "split mind." Although Bleuler based his conception of schizophrenia on Kraepelin's work, he saw it as being characterized by "primary symptoms" such as autism (by which he meant turning inward), blocking of thoughts, and loose associations (vague connections between thoughts).[7] Bleuler believed that hallucinations and delusions were "secondary symptoms" resulting from the primary thought disturbance.

Both Kraepelin and Bleuler believed that the condition each described (or invented) was caused by a disease process triggered by an inherited predisposition (*Anlage*). Lacking any twin, adoption, or molecular genetic data, Kraepelin believed that his dementia praecox concept required a "hereditary predisposition" (which he also referred to as "hereditary taint") in roughly 50–70 percent of the cases.[8] For his schizophrenia, Bleuler believed that "great importance should be attached to *hereditary burdening*," based on his observation that "among the direct ancestors of the patients, psychoses, especially schizophrenia, are much more numerous than with the healthy."[9] We will see in Chapter 3 that in this era, though not so today, it was taken for granted that a condition "running in the family" did so because of heredity.

Psychiatric Descriptions of Schizophrenia

For contemporary psychiatry and its psychiatric genetics subfield (discussed below), schizophrenia is "a severe mental disorder with a lifetime risk of about 1%, characterized by hallucinations, delusions and cognitive deficits, with heritability estimated at up to 80%," or "a heritable brain illness with unknown pathogenic mechanisms."[10]

According to the U.S. National Institute of Mental Health (NIMH), "Schizophrenia is a chronic and severe mental disorder that affects how a person thinks, feels, and behaves. People with schizophrenia may seem like they have lost touch with reality... . The symptoms can be very disabling." Schizophrenia's "positive symptoms," according to the NIMH, include "hallucinations," "delusions," "thought disorders (unusual or dysfunctional ways of thinking)," and "movement disorders (agitated body movements)." Schizophrenia's "negative symptoms" include "flat affect (reduced expression of emotions via facial expression or voice tone)," "reduced feelings of pleasure in everyday life," "difficulty beginning and sustaining activities," and "reduced speaking."[11] In the American Psychiatric Association's (APA) Diagnostic and Statistical Manual (commonly known as the "DSM"), which lists psychiatry's mental disorders and their diagnostic criteria, only some of these symptoms are necessary to diagnose someone with schizophrenia.

Mainstream sources report the worldwide average "lifetime risk" for schizophrenia as .05–1 percent, meaning that roughly 1 in every 100–200 people will be diagnosed with the condition at some point in their lives.[12]

The schizophrenia population prevalence, which refers to the percentage of diagnosed people in a population at a given time, ranges widely across the world from 2 per 1,000 to 17 per 1,000. The U.S. prevalence rate is about 8 per 1,000.[13] Schizophrenia prevalence is slightly higher among men than among women.[14] People living in poverty, relative poverty, and people of color are diagnosed more often than people not falling into these categories.[15] Although biological psychiatry offers various explanations for this finding, the stress of living in poverty and experiencing oppression, in addition to an institutionalized tendency to more often place the "schizophrenia" label on the poor, are the most likely explanations.

Criticism of the "Schizophrenia" Concept

There is a long history of controversy surrounding the schizophrenia concept, and of medical approaches to it. I will explore these controversies more in the final chapter. I am in general agreement with those who question the schizophrenia diagnosis/concept, and who argue that the term *psychosis* better describes people's experiences and behavior. I use the term "schizophrenia" in this book without quotation marks mainly to render the text less cumbersome. As critical psychiatrist R. D. Laing once remarked at an academic conference, "I am unhappy about using the term schizophrenia at all. But it would be somewhat whimsical to eliminate it from my vocabulary, since it is on the lips of so many."[16]

Psychiatric Genetics

The *psychiatric genetics* field was established in Germany in the early part of the 20th century. The Department of Genealogy and Demography at the German Institute for Psychiatric Research (Deutsche Forschungsanstalt für Psychiatrie) was founded in 1917 in Munich. In 1924, it was integrated into the Kaiser Wilhelm Society.[17] During the interwar period, psychiatric geneticists of the German "Munich School" performed family and twin studies to establish the genetic basis of psychiatric disorders, and socially disapproved behavior such as criminality. They believed that family and twin studies showed definitively that heredity played a major role. Their primary goal was to promote the eugenic program (called *Rassenhygiene* or "racial hygiene" in Germany) of curbing the reproduction of people they viewed as carrying the "hereditary taint of mental illness," by sterilization or other means.[18]

The founder of the psychiatric genetics field was the Swiss-German psychiatrist Ernst Rüdin (1874–1952), whose work and deeds I will discuss in Chapter 3. For now, it is enough to note that Rüdin performed the first schizophrenia family study in 1916 and that he believed that schizophrenia was caused by a single recessive gene.[19]

Eugenic theories, laws, and practices, which harmed millions of people, were backed by a false set of claims (premises) based on very bad "science" and on the social prejudices of the economically powerful, who helped fund and support the eugenics movement.[20] Eugenicists claimed that hereditary influences on human behavior are paramount and that environmental influences on human behavior are inconsequential. They promoted policies attempting to curb the reproduction of people they called "hereditarily unfit," while promoting the reproduction of the "hereditarily fit."

The psychiatric genetics field fell into decline in the years after World War II after the revelations of Nazi genocide and the Holocaust, and the atrocities committed against the presumed carriers of the "hereditary taint" of mental disorders.[21] The field has made a comeback in the past few decades as biological approaches in psychiatry have become predominant, and the International Society of Psychiatric Genetics (ISPG) holds an annual "World Congress of Psychiatric Genetics" (WCPG).

Modern psychiatric geneticists continue to perform family and twin studies, and in the last 60 years or so have added adoption and molecular genetic research. In the past two decades, with improved technological tools available, the field has placed much more emphasis on molecular genetic methods. In these studies, researchers attempt to identify genes that are "associated with" or cause psychiatric conditions. Psychiatric geneticists maintain that the genetic basis of most psychiatric conditions is an established fact, in much the same way they did during Rüdin's time. They attempt to assess the influence of genetic factors on psychiatric conditions, which they often refer to as "diseases," and search for predisposing genes in the belief that this will lead to better understanding, treatment, and prevention.

The allied and overlapping field of *human behavioral genetics* (or more commonly "behavioral genetics") was founded in the 1950s and 1960s.[22] Behavioral genetics is rooted in the field of psychology, and uses family, twin, adoption, and molecular genetic studies to assess the role of genetic influences on characteristics such as IQ, personality, psychiatric disorders, criminality, and other aspects of behavior.

Genetic Counseling

Although the psychiatric genetics field no longer promotes eugenic policies by name, it does promote genetic counseling programs, which lead to the reduction of births to people it sees as being the carriers of genes for psychiatric disorders.[23] There certainly can be a eugenic aspect to genetic counseling, and many eugenicists regrouped under this banner in the early post–World War II era.[24] In a 2003 article titled "Will the Genomics Revolution Revolutionize Psychiatry," genetic researchers Kathleen Merikangas and Neil Risch stated, "The goal of genomics research is ultimately prevention, the cornerstone of public health."[25] Attempts to improve environmental conditions and other primary prevention approaches are ways to increase prevention, but for those who see schizophrenia as a genetic disorder, persuading, incentivizing, coercing, or prohibiting presumed gene carriers from reproducing is another preventative method.

Reductionism

Psychiatric genetics takes a *reductionist* approach to psychiatric conditions, which in the behavioral sciences has been defined as "the belief that human behavior can be explained by breaking it down into smaller component parts."[26] In his 2002 book *Creating Mental Illness*, sociologist Allan Horwitz described the reductionist model as "an essential aspect of biological thought":

> The biological model reduces the operation of complex wholes to the properties of their individual parts. Parts are used to explain the wholes … . In the study of human societies, this means that the group is reduced to its individual members.[27]

Although schizophrenia genetic researchers recognize a role for environmental factors, their research is based on this reductionistic approach and on the belief that to understand the condition, it is necessary to identify the smallest component parts such as genes and neurotransmitters, with little regard to a person's social context. *Genetic (biological) determinism* is the argument that most human mental characteristics are determined at conception by hereditary factors passed from parent to offspring, largely but not entirely unaffected by environmental factors.

Presidential Statement

This extract from a 2022 online "Current Presidential Vision" statement by ISPG President Jordan Smoller illustrates how the field views itself:

> The field of psychiatric genetics has seen transformative progress over the past decade. It has emerged as a leading frontier in human genetics, with a robust tradition of genetic epidemiology, the successful identification of hundreds of genomic loci associated with a broad spectrum of psychiatric disorders, and a growing understanding of the genetic architecture of some of the most challenging and impactful phenotypes in all of biomedicine. This progress has been due in large part to the extraordinarily collaborative efforts of scientists and trainees across the world.[28]

This is an eloquent description of the psychiatric genetics field, but does eloquent language serve to describe real and important discoveries, or to compensate for a lack of such discoveries?

In this book, I will argue that major psychiatric genetic claims and assumptions as they relate to schizophrenia are either false or highly questionable, and that the field's comeback from the ashes of World War II was based not on real or meaningful discoveries, but on poorly performed and misinterpreted studies, accompanied by strong doses of hype. As I discussed earlier, these problems go well beyond the schizophrenia diagnosis and into other areas of psychiatry and behavior, where similar research methods are used. This is an important message of this book. I will now look more closely at how the causes of schizophrenia have been conceptualized.

Schizophrenia as a "Multifactorial Complex Disorder"

For much of the 20th century, psychiatric genetic researchers believed that schizophrenia was caused by a single gene, or by a few genes of large effect, and early molecular genetic studies focused on finding such genes (see Chapter 2). By the 1990s, mainstream researchers abandoned the search for a major causative single gene because the evidence did not support this idea, and they now view schizophrenia and other psychiatric conditions as "multifactorial complex disorders" caused by a complex interaction of multiple genes and multiple environmental risk factors. The authors of mainstream publications usually assign a major role to genetic factors and suggest that environmental factors, while necessary, are not well understood. This helps maintain focus and emphasis on the presumed genetic factors.

The predisposition-stress/multifactorial complex disorder position, as well as the "biopsychosocial" model, has been very successful in supporting the idea that psychiatric disorders have an important genetic basis. The *biopsychosocial model* is the broad view that "biological, psychological and social factors causally influence" mental health and psychiatric conditions.[29] Psychologist Mary Boyle, a critic of schizophrenia genetic research and the author of *Schizophrenia: A Scientific Delusion?* observed that the predisposition-stress model seems inclusive and reasonable in the sense that "who could deny that biological and psychological or social factors interact?" At the same time, the model

> firmly maintains the primacy of biology, not least through word order, and potentially de-emphasizes the environment by making it look as if the "stress" part of the vulnerability-stress model consists of ordinary stresses which most of us would cope with, but which overwhelm only "vulnerable" people.[30]

Boyle noted that by "inserting an unspecified innate vulnerability between the person and their environment, the claimed vulnerability and not the environment becomes the focus of concern."[31]

Environmental Factors

As reviewed by John Read in several chapters in the 2013 second edition of *Models of Madness: Psychological, Social and Biological Approaches to Psychosis*, since the turn of the 21st century many studies have linked schizophrenia and other psychotic conditions to childhood adversities such as having experienced bullying, emotional abuse, incest, neglect, parental loss, physical abuse, and sexual abuse—adversities that clinicians who work with people diagnosed with psychotic disorders are well aware of.[32] Read also reviewed the evidence linking schizophrenia and psychotic disorders to social factors such as poverty, racism, migratory stress, and urbanicity. He concluded, "There is ample evidence that inequality, deprivation and discrimination, filtered through their social and personal meanings, are key causal factors in psychosis."[33] Since then, other studies have supported a link between schizophrenia/psychosis and childhood adversity and trauma.[34]

In support of the "Traumagenic Neurodevelopmental" (TN) model of psychosis, in 2014 Read, Roar Fosse, and their colleagues summarized research findings pointing to significant risk factors for psychosis, which include

> mother's health, nutrition and stress during pregnancy, being the product of an unwanted pregnancy, early loss of parents via death or abandonment, separation of parents, witnessing interparental violence, dysfunctional parenting (often intergenerational), war trauma, rape or physical assaults as an adult, racial or other forms of discrimination, heavy marijuana use in early adolescence, and poverty.[35]

Read and colleagues described processes through which childhood adversities may lead to psychotic experiences later in life as attachment disruption, dissociation, dysfunctional cognitive processes, psychodynamic defenses, problematic coping responses, impaired access to social support, behavioral sensitization, and revictimization.[36] Read commented that "the idea that bad things happening in childhood can drive you crazy is not ... controversial in the real world beyond biological psychiatry."[37]

In a schizophrenia adoption study I will discuss briefly in Chapter 6, Pekka Tienari and colleagues believed they had confirmed a genetic influence (a conclusion I challenge in that chapter and elsewhere[38]), but they also found that

> none of the 49 [adopted-away] offspring of schizophrenic mothers who were reared in a healthy family environment or in a mildly disturbed family environment have become schizophrenic or borderline, while 37.2 percent have become psychotic or borderline when reared in a severely disturbed adoptive family.[39]

This finding provides additional evidence that the family environment can play an important role in causing or preventing schizophrenia and psychosis. In addition, we will see in Chapter 6 that in the Danish-American adoption studies, adopted children placed in the homes of Danish couples screened for mental health and economic stability reduced by over 60 percent the chance that these children, as adults, would be diagnosed with a "schizophrenia spectrum disorder."

If trauma and psychologically unhealthy family, social, and political arrangements are indeed the main factors underlying emotional problems and psychiatric diagnoses such as schizophrenia, depression, and many others, then focusing on genetics and the brain diverts society's attention from focusing on these areas. While mainstream psychiatric researchers and others worry about the "societal burden of mental disorders,"[40] from the perspective of seeing many aspects of Western society as causing psychological harm to people, much human psychological distress and dysfunction can be characterized as *the mental burden of societal disorders*.

Further Problems with Genetic Explanations of Schizophrenia

Most Diagnosed People Have No Family History of Psychosis

According to the 2013, Fifth Edition of the DSM (DSM-5), "most individuals who have been diagnosed with [schizophrenia] have no family history of psychosis."[41] In a 2006 Swedish study based on a population-based cohort of 7,739,202 individuals, Paul Lichtenstein and colleagues found that in families in which one member was diagnosed with schizophrenia, in more than 96 percent of these families, there were no other similarly diagnosed family members.[42]

In his 1991 book *Schizophrenia Genesis: The Origins of Madness*, leading schizophrenia genetics authority Irving Gottesman (1930–2016) wrote,

> The vast majority of schizophrenics will have *neither* parent who is overtly schizophrenic—some 89 percent—and will have *neither* parents nor siblings who are affected—some 81 percent. Furthermore, a sizable majority—about 63 percent—will have *negative* family histories—that is, "clean pedigrees"—even allowing for such first-degree relatives as children and such second-degree relatives as nieces and nephews.[43]

Although Gottesman was a leading supporter of psychiatric genetic theories of schizophrenia for five decades, it is difficult to imagine schizophrenia as a genetically based disorder when about two-thirds of people carrying the diagnosis have no family history of it.

Low Reproduction Rates

People diagnosed or labeled with schizophrenia often do not have children. The persistence of a "hereditary disorder" in which the gene carriers reproduce at low rates does not seem possible. Biological psychiatrist E. Fuller Torrey described the "schizophrenia paradox–the continuing existence of schizophrenia despite a low fertility rate and a high mortality rate." He observed that "between 1830 and 1950 the vast majority of individuals with severe schizophrenia were confined to mental hospitals, unable to procreate. Yet during those same years the prevalence of schizophrenia appeared to increase."[44] Although most people labeled "schizophrenic" in Nazi Germany tragically and criminally were either sterilized or killed by the regime and its willing accomplices in science and medicine (see Chapter 3), studies show, contrary to genetic predictions, a high incidence rate of new schizophrenia cases in Germany.[45] As Read and Eleanor Longden wrote, "this atrocity provided proof against the very reasoning used to instigate it."[46]

In support of genetic theories and the idea that schizophrenia is a medical illness, psychiatry has claimed that schizophrenia prevalence and incidence is similar throughout the world. In *Schizophrenia Genesis*, for example, Gottesman felt "safe to conclude that the incidence of schizophrenia in most human populations around the world today is rather similar."[47] In addition to the differing prevalence rates I have already noted, John Read has shown that schizophrenia prevalence and incidence studies do not support this claim, and that recent psychiatry textbooks have finally abandoned this "uniform prevalence myth."[48] The uniform prevalence claim was always questionable because few medical disorders, genetic or otherwise, have similar incidence or prevalence rates across all populations

Is "Schizophrenia" a Valid Disorder that Can Be Reliably Identified?

Establishing both the reliability and validity of a diagnostic concept such as schizophrenia is a prerequisite for any attempt to search for genes or genetic influences. Reliability in psychiatry refers to the ability of psychiatrists or others to consistently agree on who should be given a diagnosis. "If researchers can't agree on who has 'schizophrenia,'" Read pointed out, "then the supposed properties of 'schizophrenia' cannot be evaluated."[49] Even if a concept can be reliably identified, it doesn't mean that the concept is valid. For example, reliable criteria were once used to identify witches, but this does not mean that witches existed.

Validity refers to whether a diagnostic concept is a meaningful biological entity, with natural boundaries that separate it from other diagnoses. In their 2013 book *Mad Science: Psychiatric Coercion, Diagnosis, and Drugs*, professors of social work Stuart Kirk, Tomi Gomory, and David Cohen questioned the validity of psychiatric disorders. "To state that a mental illness is a valid concept (that it truly identifies a phenomenon of nature)," they wrote, "means that some body of *evidence* has been amassed according to the guidelines of a specific biomedical *theory*, and then has survived rigorous tests devised upon the notion that the specific theory might be false." They emphasized that simply "describing a set of behaviors and labeling them as pathological symptoms never establishes the validity of an illness," because "the criteria merely describe what is claimed a priori to be an illness."[50] As another writer observed, DSM diagnostic criteria "can't tell us whether the list of symptoms, no matter how reliable, constitutes a disease."[51]

Many critics of psychiatry have argued that psychiatric disorders are not reliable or valid illnesses, but instead describe people's sometimes meaningful and understandable psychological responses to having experienced adverse events and environments, or are socially disapproved behaviors or responses to oppression that psychiatry labels "mental (medical) disorders."

The noted psychiatrist and medical geneticist Lionel Penrose wrote in 1968, "The study of the genetics of schizophrenia is unsatisfactory from almost every point of view," with the first reason being that "there is no certainty that the condition can be defined or even recognized."[52] This position found support in the "Cross-National Project for the Study of the Diagnosis of Mental Disorders in the United States and the United Kingdom" in the late 1960s, which assessed the diagnostic practices of New York and London psychiatrists. After finding "that the American psychiatrists, in general, applied the diagnosis of schizophrenia to a much wider variety of clinical conditions than did their British colleagues,"[53] the study concluded, "The evidence presented from this series of studies strongly indicates that the diagnoses routinely made in clinical practice should not be relied upon in epidemiological studies."[54] In Chapter 6, we will see that the famous Danish-American schizophrenia adoption studies were based on psychiatric diagnoses made during this era.

Although psychiatry claims to have subsequently solved its reliability and validity problems with the development of DSM-III-and-after "operationalized diagnostic criteria," much doubt remains.[55] According to the 1980 DSM-III, a person could be diagnosed with schizophrenia by exhibiting only "markedly illogical thinking" associated with "blunted, flat, or inappropriate affect," with a "deterioration from a previous level of functioning in such areas as work, social relations, and self-care" for at least six months.[56] These criteria could be used to diagnose someone with depression, depending on how one defines the subjective DSM term "markedly illogical thinking." Cognitive-behavioral therapy (CBT) theorists point out that we all engage in illogical thinking from time to time.

The criteria for diagnosing schizophrenia remain vague and subjective. Reliability remains low, and is even decreasing.[57] As Read has shown, there are 15 ways that two people can meet the DSM criteria for schizophrenia without sharing any symptoms in common.[58] "The people studied by one researcher," as Read put it, "may have little in common with those being studied by another researcher."[59] Psychiatrist Allen Frances, former Chair of the 1994 DSM-IV Task Force, wrote in 2011 that "schizophrenia is admittedly a flawed construct with limited descriptive and explanatory power. It is ... wildly heterogeneous with dozens of different presentations and probably hundreds of different causes (none of them known)."[60] One way psychiatry tries to overcome the validity problem is to assert that schizophrenia is a brain disease, which is the topic of the next section.

Brain Disease Theories

Biological psychiatrist Nancy Andreasen wrote in a 1998 edition of the *American Journal of Psychiatry* she edited that American psychiatry may need "to organize a reverse Marshall Plan so that the Europeans can save American science by helping us figure out who really has schizophrenia or what schizophrenia really is."[61] This well-known psychiatrist's stunning admission in American psychiatry's leading journal that her field doesn't know what schizophrenia is, or who has it and who doesn't, did not prevent her from claiming in her 2001 book *Brave New Brain: Conquering Mental Illness in the Era of the Genome* that "schizophrenia" is a "brain/ mind disease" caused by an "'invisible lesion' that cannot be seen with the naked eye or under a microscope."[62] Two decades later, leading psychiatric genetic researcher Kenneth Kendler recognized, "Despite years of research, we cannot explain or directly observe the pathophysiologies of major mental health disorders that we could use to define essential features." The authors of a 2022 analysis, which included one of the most influential brain scientists in the world, concluded, "despite three decades of intense neuro-imaging research, we still lack a neurobiological account for any psychiatric condition."[63]

There are no laboratory tests for schizophrenia. A diagnosis is made on the basis of family history, personal history, behavior, speech, self-report, and the reports of others.[64] "Schizophrenia," wrote critical psychiatrist Joanna Moncrieff and Hugh Middleton, "remains a condition that is defined by unusual talk and behaviour."[65] According to Torrey, psychiatry needs, but does not have, "objective measures for diagnosis, such as laboratory tests of blood and cerebrospinal fluid. Until that time, criteria for the diagnosis of schizophrenia will continue to be debated and will require skilled clinical judgement."[66] What remains unclear is why "skilled clinical judgement" is needed to diagnose someone with schizophrenia if DSM "checking the boxes" criteria are valid, or what knowledge lies behind these judgments. Earlier speculation that schizophrenia is caused by a genetically linked deficiency of the neurotransmitter dopamine (the "dopamine hypothesis") has largely gone by the wayside, a fate similar to the unsupported "serotonin theory" of major depression.[67]

Boyle argued that in the absence of direct evidence, psychiatry must resort to "smoke and mirrors" tactics to support its brain disease claims.[68] John Read quoted a passage from the 1913 edition of Kraepelin's textbook, where Kraepelin wrote that the causes of dementia praecox "are at the present time still wrapped in impenetrable darkness." Read commented that the key phrase is "at the present time," which has "been used ever since by researchers forever on the verge of finding the biological cause of schizophrenia."[69] It should also be noted that a brain disease, like other medical conditions, can be caused by non-genetic factors.

Another factor to consider is that discovering changes in the brain correlated with a schizophrenia diagnosis does not mean that brain malfunction is the cause, and many researchers confuse cause and effect. People's experiences can modify brain anatomy and function, and the use of neuroleptic ("anti-psychotic") drugs has been shown to cause brain shrinkage and other abnormalities.[70]

The claim that schizophrenia is a brain disease is sometimes cited in support of the genetic position, and the claim that schizophrenia is rooted in genetics is sometimes cited in support of the brain disease position. R. D. Laing pointed out that because these two disputed ideas might both be wrong, one cannot be used to support the other: "These two theories do not...as is claimed, reciprocally validate each other. Rubbing two phantom flints produces only the illusion of fire."[71]

The Replication Crisis in Behavioral Research

Scientific research is in a state of crisis, and this crisis has much relevance to the body of schizophrenia genetic research I will examine in this book. It is known as the *replication crisis* (also known as the "replicability crisis" or the "reproducibility crisis"), meaning a crisis brought about by the discovery that some key findings across various scientific fields were probably non-findings resulting from research that was poorly performed, manipulated to match researcher or funding source expectations, or even fraudulent, and this may be only the tip of the iceberg.[72] In the field of psychology, where the crisis began, undetected "questionable research practices" (QRPs) appear to be common,[73] and the field has been shaken in recent years by study retractions (e.g., the work of the famous psychologist H. J. Eysenck),[74] "p-hacking,"[75] and even fabricated research.[76] And as I have shown elsewhere, in the famous "Minnesota Study of Twins Reared Apart" IQ study the researchers had to suppress and omit the IQ correlations produced by their designated control group to arrive at desired conclusions.[77]

A 2015 article was published in *Science* by the Open Science Collaboration, who undertook a "large-scale, collaborative effort to obtain an initial estimate of the reproducibility of psychological science." They found that although 97 percent of the original psychological studies in their sample had reported statistically significant results (p < .05), only 36 percent could be independently replicated at a statistically significant level.[78] Some reasons for this result, according to the investigators, included "selective reporting, selective analysis, and insufficient specification of the conditions necessary or sufficient to obtain the results."[79]

Problems in psychological research were the subject of cognitive neuroscientist Chris Chambers' 2017 book *The Seven Deadly Sins of Psychology: A Manifesto for Reforming the Culture of Scientific Practice*, and of psychologist Stuart Ritchie's 2020 book *Science Fictions: How Fraud, Bias, Negligence, and Hype Undermine the Search for Truth*.[80] The problems these authors described are not limited to psychology and occur in many other areas of scientific research.[81]

Although many behavioral science researchers did not and do not engage in such practices, most of the genetic research I will review in this book was performed and published in an era in which many of the research practices that led to the replication crisis apparently were common. Publications appearing in peer-reviewed behavioral science journals often were presented as neatly packaged articles, with little prior record of researchers' intended methods, assumptions, definitions, comparisons, and decision-making processes.[82]

The conclusions people arrive at are often influenced by *confirmation bias*, which is the tendency for people to search for, interpret, favor, and recall information in a way that confirms their preexisting beliefs or theories. We are all subject to confirmation biases. Problems mainly arise when people and fields deny its influence.

Chambers described several major problem areas in the research/publication process in psychology and other fields.[83] One of these problems is *hidden flexibility*, which refers to researchers' behind-the-scenes ability to change various aspects of their study after reviewing their data, but before submitting their paper for publication.

Both Chambers and Ritchie called for the establishment of research *preregistration*, where investigators would have the option or be required to submit their research rationale, hypotheses, design and analytic strategy, and planned data-collection stop point to a journal for peer review *before* collecting and analyzing data (more on this point below).[84]

Questionable Research Practices (QRPs)

Behavioral scientist Leslie John and colleagues introduced the *questionable research practices* (QRP) concept in 2012. "Although cases of overt scientific misconduct have received significant media attention recently," they wrote, "questionable research practices (QRPs) … increase the likelihood of finding support for a false hypothesis." QRPs "are often questionable as opposed to blatantly improper," and "offer considerable latitude for rationalization and self-deception."[85]

John and colleagues listed ten QRPs, which I reproduce here. (1) "Failing to report all of a study's dependent measures," (2) "Deciding whether to collect more data after looking to see whether the results were significant," (3) "Failing to report all of a study's conditions," (4) "Stopping collecting data earlier than planned because one found the result that one had been looking for," (5) "'Rounding off' a p value (e.g., reporting that a p value of .054 is less than .05)," (6) "Selectively reporting studies that 'worked,'" (7) "Deciding whether to exclude data after looking at the impact of doing so on the results," (8) "Reporting an unexpected finding as having been predicted from the start," (9) "Claiming that results are unaffected by demographic variables…when one is actually unsure (or knows that they [are])," and (10) "Falsifying data."[86]

To this list I would add an additional QRP relevant to the twin, adoption, and molecular genetic research I will examine in this book: claiming that conclusions are unaffected by a reliance on assumptions one is unsure of, or suspects are false. Where we decide to draw the line between QRPs and fraud is a matter of opinion.

P-hacking

A major aspect of QRPs is *p-hacking*, which describes the practice of consciously or unconsciously manipulating data to produce results that fall below the conventional .05 level of statistical significance. This means that there was less than a 5 percent probability that the finding occurred by chance. P-hacking is a set of practices researchers use to turn non-findings into claimed findings.[87] As described by evolutionary biologist Megan Head and colleagues in 2015, the "widespread" practice of p-hacking occurs "when researchers collect or select data or statistical analyses until nonsignificant results become significant," which is sometimes achieved by continuing to collect data past the planned stop point if significant comparisons are not found, and then stopping data collection at the point where < .05 statistical significance is achieved (John and colleagues' QRPs #2 and #4). Ritchie described the practice of "not setting the sample size beforehand" as allowing "researchers to continue collecting data and testing it, collecting data and testing it, again and again in an open-ended way until they get their desired p < 0.05."[88]

Another p-hacking method mentioned by Head and colleagues "occurs when researchers try out several statistical analyses and/or data eligibility specifications and then selectively report those that produce significant results" (John and colleagues' QRP #6).[89] Many investigators of previous eras engaging in what we now call p-hacking practices may not have seen anything particularly wrong with the practice, because apparently it was part of the accepted culture in which they operated.[90]

HARKing and Fishing Expeditions

Two other QRPs are *HARKing* and *fishing expeditions*. HARKing stands for "hypothesizing after the results are known."[91] Psychologist Norbert Kerr defined HARKing as "presenting a post hoc hypothesis in the introduction of a research report as if it were an a priori hypothesis" (John and colleagues' QRP #8).[92] In Chambers' words, "HARKing is a form of academic deception in which the experimental hypothesis...of a study is altered after analyzing the data in order to pretend that the authors predicted results that, in reality, were unexpected." Chambers wrote that HARKing helps produce the "clean and confirmatory papers that psychology journals prefer while also maintaining the illusion that the research is hypothesis driven and thus consistent with" standard hypothesis testing principles.[93] The authors of a 2017 "Manifesto for Reproducible Science" wrote that HARKing leads not to scientific discovery, but to "self-deception."[94]

A fishing expedition involves investigators searching through data to find statistically significant trends or differences, without testing a prior hypothesis. Identifying correlations and unexpected findings can be useful to help arrive at a new hypothesis, but that hypothesis must then be tested on a different set of data. As the authors of a medical textbook emphasized, a hypothesis cannot be developed and tested using the same data set:

> The scientific process requires that hypothesis development and hypothesis testing be based on *different* data sets. One data set is used to develop the hypothesis or model, which is used to make predictions, which are then tested on a new data set.[95]

Scientists generate hypotheses with existing observations and then test these hypotheses with later observations. Those arriving at conclusions by HARKing and by engaging in fishing expeditions, on the other hand, make *post*dictions created *after* reviewing their data.[96]

The Need for Research Preregistration in the Social and Behavioral Sciences

Building on calls by previous authors going back to the 1960s, which includes my own 2000 proposal co-authored by psychologist Steve Baldwin, Chambers called for the establishment of psychology research "preregistration," where investigators would be required to submit an introduction, and their proposed methods and analyses, *before* they collect their data.[97] Although "we may never be able to eliminate bias altogether from human nature," Chambers wrote, a "sure way to immunize ourselves against its consequences…is peer-reviewed study preregistration."[98] Fortunately, calls for pre-registration in the behavioral sciences are increasing. As Chambers described it,

> The essence of preregistration is that the study rationale, hypotheses, experimental methods, and analysis plan are stated publicly in advance of collecting data… . Since authors will have stated their hypotheses in advance, preregistration prevents HARKing and ensures adherence to the H-D [standard "hypothetico-deductive"] model of the scientific method … . Preregistration also prevents researchers from cherry-picking results that they believe generate a desirable narrative.[99]

The preregistration of behavioral research would greatly reduce p-hacking and other QRPs brought to light in the replication crisis. There is growing support for the *Register Reports* idea, which as described at the Center for Open Science website,

> is a publishing format that emphasizes the importance of the research question and the quality of methodology by conducting peer review

prior to data collection. High quality protocols are then provisionally accepted for publication if the authors follow through with the registered methodology... . It eliminates a variety of questionable research practices, including low statistical power, selective reporting of results, and publication bias, while allowing complete flexibility to report serendipitous findings.[100]

In the past, critics of genetic research in psychiatry didn't have a widely agreed-upon framework and language to explain how unsound research in this field is performed, published, and validated. The QRP and p-hacking concepts now provide such a framework. In the chapters to come I will show that a reliance on false assumptions and the use of QRPs are common in schizophrenia genetic research, and only through the use of such practices has the widespread acceptance of schizophrenia as a genetic medical-type illness been sustained.

Summary and Conclusions

In this chapter, I listed the most important research methods used to support the "high heritability" of schizophrenia and psychosis, which are the main areas of this book's focus: family studies, twin studies, adoption studies, and molecular genetic studies. I then showed that the "genetics of schizophrenia" question has much larger implications relating to the nature-nurture debate and the question of what it means to be human. I discussed the history of the schizophrenia concept and the controversies surrounding it, and I described the field of psychiatric genetics. I then explored the evidence in favor of environmental (non-genetic) causes, and noted several aspects of schizophrenia that are difficult to explain on genetic grounds. This was followed by an examination of reductionistic versus social understandings of psychological distress and dysfunction. Although psychiatry has marshaled evidence it claims supports brain disease and genetic theories of causation, both are disputed theories. I ended the chapter with a discussion of the ongoing "replication crisis" in the behavioral sciences and elsewhere, and its relevance to a proper understanding of the schizophrenia genetic research I will examine in the following chapters.

In 1980, sociologist Howard Taylor described what he called the "IQ Game" in psychology and behavioral genetics, by which he meant IQ-genetic researchers' "use of assumptions that are implausible as well as arbitrary to arrive at some numerical value for the genetic heritability of human IQ scores on the grounds that no heritability calculations could be made without benefit of such assumptions."[101] In the chapters to come I will explore the question of whether schizophrenia genetic research is definitive, as most textbooks report, or whether it is better understood as "the schizophrenia game."

Notes

1 Anonymous (2003), Scientific Breakthrough of the Year: The Runners-Up, *Science, 302,* 2039–2045, p. 2039. https://doi.org/10.1126/science.302.5653 .2039

2 Farrell et al. (2015), Evaluating Historical Candidate Genes for Schizophrenia, *Molecular Psychiatry, 20, 555–562*, p. 560. https://doi.org/10.1038/mp.2015.16

3 Leo, J. (2016), The Search for Schizophrenia Genes, *Issues in Science and Technology, 32*(2), 68–71. https://issues.org/the-search-for-schizophrenia -genes/

4 Boyle, M., & Johnstone, L. (2020), *A Straight Talking Introduction to the Power Threat Meaning Framework: An Alternative to Psychiatric Diagnosis,* Monmouth, UK: PCCS Books, p. 105.

5 Arieti, S. (1974), *Interpretation of Schizophrenia* (2nd ed.), New York: Basic Books.

6 Arieti, 1974.

7 Bleuler, E. (1950), *Dementia Praecox or the Group of Schizophrenias,* New York: International Universities Press (original German edition published in 1911).

8 Kraepelin, E. (2018), *Dementia Praecox and Paraphrenia,* London: Forgotten Books (original English translation published in 1919), pp. 232–233.

9 Bleuler, E. (2018), *Textbook of Psychiatry,* London: Forgotten Books (original English translation published in 1924), p. 441.

10 International Schizophrenia Consortium (2009), Common Polygenic Variation Contributes to Risk of Schizophrenia and Bipolar Disorder, *Nature, 460,* 748–752, p. 748. https://doi.org/10.1038/nature08185; Sekar et al. (2016), Schizophrenia Risk from Complex Variation of Complement Component 4, *Nature, 530,* 177–183, p. 177. https://doi.org/10.1038/nature16549

11 https://www.nimh.nih.gov/health/topics/schizophrenia

12 Glatt, S. J., Faraone, S. V., & Tsuang, M. T. (2019), *Schizophrenia: The Facts* (4th ed.), Oxford, UK: Oxford University Press.

13 Torrey, E. F. (2019), *Surviving Schizophrenia: A Family Manual* (7th ed.), New York: Harper Perennial, p. 373.

14 Jauhar, S., Johnstone, M., & McKenna, P. J. (2022), Schizophrenia, *Lancet, 399,* 473–486. https://doi.org/10.1016/S0140-6736(21)01730-X

15 Hollingshead, A. B., & Redlich, F. C. (1958), *Social Class and Mental Illness: A Community Study,* New York: John Wiley & Sons; Read, J. Johnstone, L., & Taitimu, M. (2013), Psychosis, Poverty and Ethnicity, in J. Read & J. Dillon (Eds.), *Models of Madness: Psychological, Social and Biological Approaches to Psychosi* (2nd ed., pp. 191–209), London: Routledge.

16 Laing, R. D. (1967), The Study of Family and Social Contexts in Relation to the Origin of Schizophrenia, in J. Romano (Ed.), *The Origins of Schizophrenia: Proceedings of the First Rochester International Conference on Schizophrenia, March 29–31, 1967* (pp. 139–146), New York: Excerpta Medica Foundation, p. 139.

17 Ritter, H. J., & Roelcke, V. (2005), Psychiatric Genetics in Munich and Basel between 1925 and 1945: Programs-Practices-Cooperative Arrangements, *Osiris (2nd Ser.), 20,* 263–288. https://doi.org/10.1086/649421

18 Joseph, J., & Wetzel, N. (2013), Ernst Rüdin: Hitler's Racial Hygiene Mastermind, *Journal of the History of Biology, 46,* 1–30. https://doi.org/10 .1007/s10739-012-9344-6; Roelcke, V. (2019), Eugenic Concerns, Scientific Practices: International Relations in the Establishment of Psychiatric Genetics in Germany, Britain, the USA and Scandinavia, *c.*1910–60. *History of Psychiatry, 30,* 19–37. https://doi.org/10.1177/0957154X18808666.

19 Rüdin, E. (1916), *Zur Vererbung und Neuentstehung der Dementia Praecox [On the Heredity and New Development of Dementia Praecox]*, Berlin: Springer Verlag OHG.

20 Black, E. (2003), *War Against the Weak: Eugenics and America's Campaign to Create a Master Race*, New York: Four Walls Eight Windows.

21 Joseph & Wetzel, 2013; Lifton, R. J. (1986), *The Nazi Doctors*, New York: Basic Books; Müller-Hill, B. (1998), *Murderous Science*, Plainview, NY: Cold Spring Harbor Laboratory Press (original English version published in 1988); Proctor, R. N. (1988), *Racial Hygiene: Medicine under the Nazis*, Cambridge, MA: Harvard University Press.

22 Fuller, J. L., & Thompson, W. R. (1960), *Behavior Genetics*, New York: John Wiley & Sons.

23 Hoge, S. K., & Appelbaum, P. S. (2008), Ethical, Legal, and Social Implications of Psychiatric Genetics and genetic counseling, in J. W. Smoller, B. R. Sheidley, & M. T. Tsuang (Eds.), *Psychiatric Genetics: Applications in Clinical Practice* (pp. 255–276), Washington, DC: American Psychiatric Publishing; Faraone, S. V., Tsuang, M. T., & Tsuang, D. W. (1999), *Genetics of Mental Disorders*, New York: Guilford.

24 Paul, D. B. (1998), *The Politics of Heredity: Essays on Eugenics, Biomedicine, and the Nature-Nurture Debate*, Albany, NY: State University of New York Press.

25 Merikangas, K. R., & Risch, N. (2003), Will the Genomics Revolution Revolutionize Psychiatry?, *American Journal of Psychiatry, 160*, 625–635, p. 632. https://doi.org/10.1176/appi.ajp.160.4.625

26 https://www.simplypsychology.org/reductionism.html

27 Horwitz, A. V. (2002), *Creating Mental Illness*, Chicago: University of Chicago Press, p. 135.

28 https://ispg.net/about-us/message-from-the-president/

29 Williamson, S. (2022), The Biopsychosocial Model: Not Dead, But in Need of Revival, *BJ Psych Bulletin*, 1–3, p. 1. https://doi.org/10.1192/bjb.2022.29

30 Boyle, M. (2002), It's All Done with Smoke and Mirrors. Or, How to Create the Illusion of a Schizophrenic Brain Disease, *Clinical Psychology, 12*, 9–16. http://www.critpsynet.freeuk.com/Boyle.htm

31 Boyle, M. (2007), The Problem with Diagnosis, *The Psychologist, 20*, 290–292, p. 291. https://thepsychologist.bps.org.uk/volume-20/edition-5/diagnosis-special-issue-part-1-2

32 Read, J. (2013), Childhood Adversity and Psychosis, in J. Read & J. Dillon (Eds.), *Models of Madness: Psychological, Social and Biological Approaches to Psychosis* (2nd ed., pp. 249–275), London: Routledge; Read, J. Johnstone, L., & Taitimu, M. (2013), Psychosis, Poverty and Ethnicity, in J. Read & J. Dillon (Eds.), *Models of Madness: Psychological, Social and Biological Approaches to Psychosis* (2nd ed., pp. 191–209), London: Routledge.

33 Read et al., 2013, Psychosis, Poverty and Ethnicity, p. 205.

34 Inyang et al. (January 21, 2022), The Role of Childhood Trauma in Psychosis and Schizophrenia: A Systematic Review, *Cureus 14*(1), e21466. https://doi.org/10.7759/cureus.21466; Misiak et al. (2022), Neurodevelopmental Aspects of Adverse Childhood Experiences in Psychosis: Relevance of the Allostatic Load Concept, *Psychoneuroendocrinology*. Advance online publication. https://doi.org/10.1016/j.psyneuen.2022.105850; Popovic et al. (2019), Childhood Trauma in Schizophrenia: Current Findings and Research Perspectives, *Frontiers in Neuroscience, 13*, 1–14. https://doi.org/10.3389/fnins.2019.00274

35 Read, J., Fosse, R., Moskowitz, A., & Perry, B. (2014), The Traumagenic Neurodevelopmental Model of Psychosis Revisited, *Neuropsychiatry, 4*, 65–79, p. 66. https://doi.org/10.2217/NPY.13.89

36 Read et al., 2014.
37 Read, J., 2013, Childhood Adversity and Psychosis, p. 253.
38 Joseph, 2004.
39 Tienari et al. (1987), Genetic and Psychosocial Factors in Schizophrenia: The Finnish Adoptive Family Study, *Schizophrenia Bulletin, 13,* 477–484, p. 483. https://doi.org/10.1093/schbul/13.3.477
40 Kessler et al. (2005), Lifetime Prevalence and Age-of-Onset Distributions of *DSM-IV* Disorders in the National Comorbidity Survey Replication, *Archives of General Psychiatry, 62,* 593–602, p. 601. https://doi.org/10.1001/archpsyc.62.6.593
41 American Psychiatric Association (2013), *Diagnostic and Statistical Manual of Mental Disorders* (5th ed.), Arlington, VA: Author [DSM-5], p. 103.
42 Lichtenstein et al. (2006), Recurrence Risks for Schizophrenia in a Swedish National Cohort, *Psychological Medicine, 36,* 1417–1425. https://doi.org/10.1017/S0033291706008385. I thank Mike Jones for bringing this study and its family recurrence rate to my attention.
43 Gottesman, I. I. (1991), *Schizophrenia Genesis: The Origins of Madness*, New York: W. H. Freeman & Company, pp. 102–103.
44 Torrey, E. F. (2019), *Surviving Schizophrenia* (7th ed.), New York: Harper Perennial, pp. 132–133.
45 Torrey, E. F., & Yolken, R. H. (2010), Psychiatric Genocide: Nazi Attempts to Eradicate Schizophrenia, *Schizophrenia Bulletin, 36,* 26–32. https://doi.org/10.1093/schbul/sbp097. See also Joseph & Wetzel, 2013; Lifton, 1986; Müller-Hill, 1998; Proctor,1988; Weiss, S. F. (2010), *The Nazi Symbiosis: Human Genetics and Politics in the Third Reich*, Chicago: University of Chicago Press
46 Longden, E., & Read, J. (2016), Social Adversity in the Etiology of Psychosis: A Review of the Evidence, *American Journal of Psychotherapy, 70,* 5–33. https://doi.org/10.1176/appi.psychotherapy.2016.70.1.5
47 Gottesman, 1991, p. 80.
48 Read, J. (2013), Biological Psychiatry's Lost Cause, in J. Read & J. Dillon (Eds.), *Models of Madness: Psychological, Social and Biological Approaches to Psychosis* (2nd ed., pp. 62–71), London: Routledge, pp. 62–63.
49 Read, J. (2013), Does "Schizophrenia" Exist? Reliability and Validity, in J. Read & J. Dillon (Eds.), *Models of Madness: Psychological, Social and Biological Approaches to Psychosis* (2nd ed., pp. 47–61), London: Routledge, p. 51.
50 Kirk, S. A., Gomory, T., & Cohen, D. (2013), *Mad Science: Psychiatric Coercion, Diagnosis, and Drugs*, New Brunswick, NJ: Transaction, pp. 164–166.
51 Greenberg, G. (2013), *The Book of Woe: The DSM and the Unmasking of Psychiatry*, New York: Blue Rider Press, pp. 42–43.
52 Penrose, L. (1968), A Critical Survey of Schizophrenia Genetics, in G. Howells (Ed.), *Modern Perspectives in World Psychiatry* (pp. 3–19), Edinburgh and London: Oliver & Boyd, p. 4.
53 Professional Staff of the United States-United Kingdom Cross National Project (1974), The Diagnosis and Psychopathology of Schizophrenia in New York and London, *Schizophrenia Bulletin, 11,* 80–102, p. 85. https://doi.org/10.1093/schbul/1.11.80
54 Professional Staff of the United States-United Kingdom Cross National Project, 1974, p. 95.
55 Boyle, M. (2002), *Schizophrenia: A Scientific Delusion?* (2nd ed.), Hove, UK: Routledge; Kirk et al., 2013; Greenberg, 2013; Kirk, S. A., & Kutchins, H. (1992), *The Selling of DSM: The Rhetoric of Science in Psychiatry* New York: Aldine De Gruyter.
56 American Psychiatric Association (1980), *Diagnostic and Statistical Manual of Mental Disorders* (3rd ed.), Washington, DC: Author, pp. 188–190.

57 Regier et al. (2013), DSM-5 Field Trials in the United States and Canada, Part II: Test-Retest Reliability of Selected Categorical Diagnoses, *American Journal of Psychiatry, 170*, 59–70. https://doi.org/10.1176/appi.ajp.2012.12070999

58 Read, J., 2013, Does "Schizophrenia" Exist?

59 Read, J., 2013, Biological Psychiatry's Lost Cause, p. 63.

60 Frances, A. (2011, July 27), The British Psychological Society Condemns DSM 5 [Web log post, *Psychology Today* "DSM5 in Distress"]. https://www.psychologytoday.com/us/blog/dsm5-in-distress/201107/the-british-psychological-society-condemns-dsm-5

61 Andreasen, N. C. (1998), Understanding Schizophrenia: A Silent Spring?, *American Journal of Psychiatry, 155*, 1657–1659, p. 1659. https://doi.org/10.1176/ajp.155.12.1657

62 Andreasen, N. C. (2001), *Brave New Brain: Conquering Mental Illness in the Era of the Genome*, Oxford: Oxford University Press, pp. 197, 209.

63 Bohannon, J. (2016, November 11th), A Computer Program Just Ranked the Most Influential Brain Scientists of the Modern Era. https://www.science.org/content/article/computer-program-just-ranked-most-influential-brain-scientists-modern-era; Kendler K. S. (2022), Potential Lessons for DSM From Contemporary Philosophy of Science, *JAMA Psychiatry, 79*, 99–100, p. 99. https://doi .org/10.1001 /jamapsychiatry.2021.3559; Nour, M. M., Liu, Y., & Dolan, R. J. (2022), Functional Neuroimaging in Psychiatry and the Case for Failing Better, *Neuron, 110*(16), 2524–2544. https://doi.org/10.1016/j.neuron.2022.07.005

64 Frances, A. (2013), *Saving Normal: An Insider's Revolt Against Out-of-Control Psychiatric Diagnosis, DSM-5, Big Pharma, and the Medicalization of Ordinary Life*, New York: William Morrow, p. 10.

65 Moncrieff & Middleton, 2009, p. 2015.

66 Torrey, 2019, p. 57.

67 Edwards et al. (2016), Evaluating the Dopamine Hypothesis of Schizophrenia in a Large-Scale Genome-Wide Association Study, *Schizophrenia Research, 176*, 136–140. https://doi.org/10.1016/j.schres.2016.06.016; Moncrieff, J. (2009), A Critique of the Dopamine Hypothesis of Schizophrenia and Psychosis, *Harvard Review of Psychiatry, 17*, 214–225. https://doi.org/10.1080/10673220902979896. Moncrieff et al. (2022), The Serotonin Theory of Depression: A Systematic Umbrella Review of the Evidence, *Molecular Psychiatry*. https://doi.org/10.1038/s41380-022-01661-0

68 Boyle, (2002), It's All Done with Smoke and Mirrors.

69 Read, J. (2013), The Invention of Schizophrenia, in J. Read & J. Dillon (Eds.), *Models of Madness: Psychological, Social and Biological Approaches to Psychosis* (2nd ed., pp. 20–33), London: Routledge, p. 23.

70 Ho et al. (2011), Long-term Antipsychotic Treatment and Brain Volumes, *Archives of General Psychiatry, 68*, 128–137. https://doi.org/10.1001/archgenpsychiatry.2010.199; Valenstein, E. S. (1988), *Blaming the Brain: The Truth About Drugs and Mental Health,* New York: The Free Press.

71 Laing, R. D. (1981), A Critique of Kallmann's and Slater's Genetic Theory of Schizophrenia, in R. Evans (Ed.), *Dialogue with R. D. Laing* (pp. 97–156), New York: Praeger, p. 97.

72 Baker, M. (2015, August 27th), Over Half of Psychology Studies Fail Reproducibility Test, *Nature,* https://doi.org/10.1038/nature.2015.18248; Open Science Collaboration (2015), Psychology: Estimating the Reproducibility of Psychological Science, *Science, 349*(6251), aac4716-1- aac47168. https://doi .org/10.1126/science.aac4716

73 John, L. K., Loewenstein, G., & Prelec, D. (2012), Measuring the Prevalence of Questionable Research Practices with Incentives for Truth Telling, *Psychological Science, 23*, 524–532. https://doi.org/10.1177/0956797611430953

74 O'Grady, C. (2020, July 15th), Misconduct Allegations Push Psychology Hero off his Pedestal, *Science*. https://www.sciencemag.org/news/2020/07/misconduct-allegations-push-psychology-hero-his-pedestal

75 Head et al. (2015), The Extent and Consequences of P-Hacking in Science, *PLoS Biology, 13*(3), e1002106. https://doi.org/10.1371/journal.pbio.1002106

76 Levelt Committee, Noort Committee, Drenth Committee (2012), *Flawed Science: The Fraudulent Research Practices of Social Psychologist Diederik Stapel*. https://www.rug.nl/about-ug/latest-news/news/archief2012/nieuwsberichten/stapel-eindrapport-eng.pdf

77 Joseph, J. (in press), A Reevaluation of the 1990 "Minnesota Study of Twins Reared Apart" IQ Study, *Human Development*. https://doi.org/10.1159/000521922. Advance online publication https://www.karger.com/Article/Pdf/521922

78 Open Science Collaboration, 2015, p. aac4716-1.

79 Open Science Collaboration, 2015, p. aac4716-1.

80 Chambers, 2017; Ritchie, S. (2020), *Science Fictions: How Fraud, Bias, Negligence, and Hype Undermine the Search for Truth*, Henry Holt and Co., Kindle Edition.

81 https://www.news-medical.net/health/The-Replication-Crisis-in-Biomedicine.aspx

82 Chambers, 2017; Joseph, J., & Baldwin, S. (2000), Four Editorial Proposals to Improve Social Sciences Research and Publication, *International Journal of Risk and Safety in Medicine, 13,* 109–116.

83 Chambers, 2017.

84 See also Joseph & Baldwin, 2000.

85 John et al., 2012, p. 524.

86 John et al., 2012, p. 525.

87 The term "p-hacking" was coined in 2014. Simonsohn, U., Nelson, L. D., & Simmons, J. P. (2014), p-Curve and Effect Size: Correcting for Publication Bias Using Only Significant Results, *Perspectives on Psychological Science, 9,* 666–681. https://doi.org/10.1177/1745691614553988

88 Ritchie, 2020, p. 134.

89 Head et al., 2015.

90 Simmons, J. P., Nelson, L. D., & Simonsohn, U. (2018), False-positive citations, *Perspectives on Psychological Science, 13,* 255–259, p. 255. https://doi.org/10.1177/1745691617698146

91 Kerr, N. L. (1998), HARKing: Hypothesizing After the Results Are Known, *Personality and Social Psychology Review, 2,* 196–217. https://doi.org/10.1207/s15327957pspr0203_4

92 Kerr, 1998, p. 197.

93 Chambers, 2017, p. 18.

94 Munafò et al. (2017), A Manifesto for Reproducible Science, *Nature Human Behaviour, 1,* 0021, p. 2. https://doi.org/10.1038/s41562-016-0021

95 Jekel et al. (2007), *Epidemiology, Biostatistics, and Preventive Medicine* (3rd ed.), Philadelphia: Saunders-Elsevier, p. 206.

96 Nosek et al. (2018), The Preregistration Revolution, *Proceedings of the National Academy of Sciences, 115*(11), 2600–2606. https://doi.org/10.1073/pnas.1708274114

97 Joseph & Baldwin, 2000.

98 Chambers, 2017, p. 174.

99 Chambers, 2017, p. 21.

100 See the Center for Open Science website https://www.cos.io/initiatives/registered-reports

101 Taylor, H. F. (1980), *The IQ Game: A Methodological Inquiry into the Heredity-Environment Controversy*, New Brunswick, NJ: Rutgers University Press, p. 7.

2 Schizophrenia Molecular Genetic Research

Running on Empty?

"Finding and Losing" Schizophrenia Genes

If predisposing genes play a role in causing schizophrenia and psychosis, molecular genetic studies should have uncovered them by now. As yet, however, causative genes have not been discovered. Considering the many "we have discovered schizophrenia gene associations" claims that have appeared in recent years based on "genome-wide association" (GWAS) and "polygenic risk score" (PRS) studies, I have chosen up front to make clear why it remains vitally important to take a closer look at the schizophrenia family, twin, and adoption studies I will evaluate in the upcoming chapters. In 2002, sociologist Peter Conrad described the pattern of gene discovery claims in psychiatry, followed by retractions and failures to replicate, as the "finding and losing" of such genes.[1] In the years since that was written, far more genes have been "found" and then "lost" than in all the years prior.

When assessing schizophrenia gene discovery claims, we should keep two main points in mind. The first is that these claims are based on "associations" between schizophrenia and genomic regions ("loci"). They are not based on the discovery of genes shown to *cause* the condition. In 2022, Thomas Insel, the biologically oriented former director of the U.S. National Institute of Mental Health, recognized that "in contrast to the mutations discovered for cancer or rare diseases, none of the genetic variants associated with mental illness can be considered causal."[2] Association means correlation, and it is well known that correlation does not imply cause. There is a strong association between vehicles traveling 50 miles per hour and vehicles having tires. This does not mean that tires *cause* a vehicle to travel 50 miles per hour.

The second point is that we must view gene discovery claims in the context of decades of similar claims that didn't hold up. Whatever mainstream investigators write *now* about their own or others' past non-replicated gene-finding reports, when these false-positive reports were being published, they often wrote of excitement, discovery, and the beginning of a new era—similar to how they now describe GWAS and PRS studies.[3] Current claims of

DOI: 10.4324/9781003293279-2

schizophrenia gene discoveries or gene associations, therefore, should be viewed with much caution and even skepticism.

The 1980s and 1990s witnessed a great expansion of molecular genetic research in psychiatry. This was followed by the publication of the initial working draft of the human genome sequence in 2001, which many people believed would lead to rapid gene discoveries in psychiatry and psychology. Psychiatric geneticists Stephen Faraone and Ming Tsuang wrote in 1999, "From the perspective of psychiatric genetics, the Human Genome Project (HGP) is an immense factory producing and refining the tools we will need to discover the genes that cause mental illness."[4] And according to genetic researchers Kathleen Merikangas and Neil Risch, writing in 2003, "Completion of the human genome project has provided an unprecedented opportunity to identify the effect of gene variants on complex phenotypes, such as psychiatric disorders."[5] But it didn't happen.[6]

Attention also has been focused on *epigenetics*, which refers to molecular mechanisms outside or around a gene that switch gene expression on and off in response to environmental events and challenges, without alteration in DNA sequence. Epigenetic changes can be passed down to the next generation independently of DNA inheritance.[7] I will not address epigenetics in this book because, although related to the environment, it is still an inside-the-body approach to understanding schizophrenia and psychosis, potentially diverting attention from needed outside-the-body approaches.

DSM-5 and Anticipated Gene Discoveries

In 2002, the American Psychiatric Association (APA) published a "speculative outline" of the then future fifth edition of its Diagnostic and Statistical Manual (DSM), which envisioned a DSM-5 practice of classifying disorders on the basis of a revised Axis I that would be "set aside for recording the patient's *genotype,* identifying symptom- or disease-related genes, resiliency genes, and genes related to therapeutic responses and side effects to specific psychotropic drugs."[8] Leaders of the APA expected that the Human Genome Project's sequencing of the human genome would lead to the rapid identification of the genes they believed underlie psychiatric disorders. However, these anticipated gene discoveries never came. The DSM-5 was finally published in 2013, and the "multiaxial diagnostic system," used in DSM III through DSM-IV-TR (1980–2013), was eliminated due to a failure—offically recognized as such by the APA in a 2013 press release—to identifty genes and biomarkers for psychiatric conditions.[9]

The "Nonreplication Curse" in Psychiatric Genetics

By 2013, Faraone was writing about the frustrating "nonreplication curse" that had plagued psychiatric molecular genetic research "for decades."[10] Five years earlier, he and his colleagues had written in an academic journal that "it is no secret that our field has published thousands of candidate gene association studies but few replicated findings."[11] But in a sense nonreplication *was* a secret because the public was being told a different story. Gene discovery claims were common and sensationalized in the popular media (examples below), leading to the public's belief that "genes for" psychiatric disorders had been discovered, when in fact no such discoveries had been made.

In a 2022 schizophrenia molecular genetic analysis, Alison Merikangas and colleagues "conducted a systematic review and synthesis of case–control studies of genome-wide gene expression in schizophrenia" published between 2000 and 2020. They found a "surprisingly small overlap in the genes reported across studies," and only one gene was found at a statistically significant elevation. This was the GBP2 gene, which was found in 5 of the 28 studies.[12]

The GWAS and PRS methods I will discuss later in this chapter are based on common (but still minority) genetic variants. These are known as *single-nucleotide polymorphisms* or "SNPs" (pronounced "snips" by those in the field). These variants, numbering in the millions and curated in an ever-growing digital catalog available to researchers, are considered "common" minority variants of genes present in at least 1 percent of the population. SNPs can be used as probabilistic markers or associative "tags" for identifying nearby genetic loci that may harbor actual causative variants when the genetic profiles of cases are compared to controls.

Another area focuses on potential rare risk variants, such as *copy number variants*, or "CNVs." Although in some ways, SNP and CNV researchers have formed rival camps, some see these approaches as complimenting each other: "These parallel lines of common and rare variant-based genetic enquiry share a common goal: increased understanding of the neuro-biology of schizophrenia."[13] Although many studies claiming CNV-schizophrenia associations have appeared in recent years, in this chapter I will focus on other more widely publicized approaches. In 2020 Jonathan Flint and Kenneth Kendler, two of the world's leading psychiatric genetic researchers, along with Ralph Greenspan wrote that the "early hope that CNVs would reflect the 'royal road' to understanding molecular genetic effects of schizophrenia has been disappointing."[14]

Justification for the gene-finding enterprise rests on the accuracy of heritability estimates derived from family resemblance patterns found in the family, twin, and adoption studies I will examine in the chapters to come. In the following section I discuss researchers' reliance on these estimates as one of many problematic areas in psychiatric molecular genetic research.

Heritability: "One of the Most Misleading Terms in the History of Science"

The production of *heritability estimates* is a key aspect of behavioral genetic and psychiatric genetic research, as these estimates both justify and guide molecular genetic research. If a heritability estimate is valid and high, for psychiatric genetic researchers this justifies the search for causative genetic variants. However, if a heritability estimate is inflated due to systematic bias, or if heritability estimates are meaningless in and of themselves (other than to indicate that genetic factors are involved in some way), then efforts to find causative genes will end up as a hugely expensive failure. Therefore, before looking more closely at schizophrenia molecular genetic research, I will review the heritability concept and highlight its major limitations.

Not a "Nature-Nurture Ratio"

In the words of critical behavioral genetic researcher Jerry Hirsch (1922–2008), "heritability" and "heredity" are "two entirely different concepts that have been hopelessly conflated." Because they sound alike, he wrote, "when we hear one of the two words, automatically we think the other." As Hirsch repeatedly pointed out, a heritability estimate is not a "nature-nurture ratio" of the relative contributions of genes and environment.[15]

Based mainly on twin study data (see Chapters 4 and 5), researchers calculate heritability estimates ranging from 0 percent to 100 percent (0.0–1.0). These estimates are frequently found in textbooks and other influential works. As Robert Plomin and other leaders of the behavioral genetics field defined it, heritability is "the proportion of phenotypic differences among individuals that can be attributed to genetic differences in a particular population."[16] For Plomin, in contrast to Hirsch, a heritability estimate indicates "how much genetics contributes to a trait."[17] Previously, in 1967 Gottesman and his frequent collaborator James Shields expressed a similar belief that heritability estimates quantify the "degree of genetic determination" of schizophrenia.[18]

The "heritability of schizophrenia" estimate is widely reported by mainstream sources at around 80 percent (see Chapter 5).[19] Table 2.1 highlights the main problems with the use of heritability estimates in human behavioral and psychiatric genetic research.

Heritability estimates in behavioral research depend on several questionable assumptions. One of these is the long-disputed assumption, seen in Table 2.1, that genetic and environmental factors are separate (additive) and do not interact. Stanford professors Marcus Feldman and Jessica Riskin objected: "We can no more unbraid genetics and environment than we can unbraid history and culture, or climate and landscape, or language and thought."[20] In a 2022 article, sociologist Nicolas Robette and colleagues examined heritability assumptions and concluded, "none of the hypotheses inherent in heritability estimates are verified in humans."[21] As psychologist David Moore and David Shenk wrote in "The Heritability Fallacy," the "term 'heritability,' as it is used today in human behavioral genetics, is one of the most misleading in the history of science."[22] This leads to a rejection of "variance explained by" descriptions of the causes of psychiatric conditions.

Table 2.1 Some Problems with Heritability Estimation in the Behavioral Sciences

1. Heritability estimates do not measure the "strength" of genetic influences on psychiatric conditions or behavioral characteristics, nor do they measure the relative importance of genetic and environmental influences.
2. Heritability estimates are based on research methods such as family, twin, and adoption studies which, to varying degrees, are unable to disentangle the potential influences of genes and environment on human behavioral differences.
3. Although heritability estimates are based on the assumption that genetic and environmental factors are separate (additive) and do not interact, they clearly do interact.
4. Even when heritability is high, or even when it is 100 percent, a simple environmental change or intervention can have an important preventative or curative impact.
5. Heritability is the property of a population, not of the characteristic or condition itself.
6. Because it is a population statistic, heritability does not describe the importance of genetic factors as they relate to an individual.
7. Heritability estimates apply only to a specific population, at a specific time, and in a specific environment. Estimates can change substantially under different environmental conditions.
8. *Within*-group heritability implies nothing about *between*-group heritability (such as between ethnic groups or between economic classes).
9. Research shows that gene expression switches on and off "epigenetically" in response to environmental events and challenges, which provides additional evidence that genetic and environmental influences are not additive but are instead interactive.
10. In general, the production of heritability estimates depends on researchers' acceptance of a string of questionable assumptions about people, genetics, behavioral characteristics, and psychiatric conditions, including the reliability and validity of psychiatric conditions.

Illustrating the "Heritability Fallacy"

I now present the example of *favism* (Glucose-6-phosphate dehydrogenase deficiency) to illustrate the fallacy of using heritability estimates to assess "how much" genes influence behaviors, psychiatric conditions, or diseases. Favism is caused by an inherited deficiency of glucose-6-phosphate. The predisposing gene is located on the X chromosome. When the carrier eats fava (broad) beans or inhales fava bean pollen, favism appears. The disease is marked by the development of hemolytic anemia. In other words, "beans and genes" are both necessary for favism to appear in humans.

Imagine that in the fictional country of "Freedonia" (from the Marx Brothers' movie *Duck Soup*), all citizens (100%) carry the favism gene. In Freedonia, 15 percent of the citizens, all of whom of course carry the gene, are exposed to fava beans and subsequently develop favism. Because all citizens carry the gene, but only some were exposed to fava beans, all favism *variation* in Freedonia is caused by environmental factors (fava bean exposure or non-exposure). The "heritability of favism" in Freedonia, therefore, is 0 percent (0.0).

Yet it would be mistaken to conclude that genes play no role in developing favism in Freedonia, or that the genetic influence is weak or irrelevant. A genetic predisposition is, in fact, a prerequisite for developing favism.

Now let's imagine that in the fictional country of "Wakanda" (from the movie *Black Panther*), all citizens (100%) eat a diet containing fava beans. In Wakanda, 15 percent of the citizens, all of whom of course eat a diet containing fava beans, carry the favism gene and subsequently develop favism. Because all citizens are exposed to fava beans but only some carry the gene, all favism *variation* in Wakanda is caused by genetic factors (carrying or not carrying the gene). The "heritability of favism" in Wakanda, therefore, is 100 percent (1.0).

Yet it would be mistaken to conclude that fava beans play no role in developing favism in Wakanda, or that fava bean exposure is irrelevant. Exposure to fava beans is, in fact, a prerequisite for developing favism. Favism heritability estimates in these two fictional countries are seen in Table 2.2.

As seen in Table 2.2, the "heritability of favism" is 0 percent in Freedonia and 100 percent in Wakanda, *even though the causes of favism are the same in both countries.* As we see, heritability estimates assess variation as opposed to cause, and do not indicate the strength or weakness of genetic influence—or by implication the strength or weakness of environmental influence. Looking at their country's favism heritability estimates, psychiatric geneticists in Freedonia would say that the genetic influence on favism is weak or nonexistent. Their colleagues in Wakanda, on the other hand, would say that the *environmental* influence on favism is weak or nonexistent. Both would be wrong because heritability estimates *do not* assess the "relative contributions of genes or environment."

It is not the task of critics to establish the "true heritability" of schizophrenia, or to demonstrate that it is zero. Both concepts, "schizophrenia"

Table 2.2 Favism in "Freedonia" and "Wakanda": Causes are the Same—Heritability Estimates Differ Dramatically

Freedonia	*Wakanda*
Percentage of Citizens Carrying the Favism Gene	Percentage of Citizens Carrying the Favism Gene
100%	15%
Percentage of Citizens Eating Fava Beans or Inhaling Fava Bean Pollen	Percentage of Citizens Eating Fava Beans or Inhaling Fava Bean Pollen
15%	100%
FAVISM HERITABILITY IN FREEDONIA	**FAVISM HERITABILITY IN WAKANDA**
0%	100%

and "heritability," are of questionable scientific validity, which casts doubt upon the claim that the "heritability of schizophrenia" qualifies as a valid or meaningful concept, whether or not genes play a role in causing the condition.

"Missing" Heritability

The "missing heritability" era began around 2008.[23] In psychiatry, the claim that "heritability is missing" is an attempt to explain the failure to identify genes that cause or predispose for psychiatric disorders by claiming that such genes exist and await discovery once better methods are found, and larger samples are obtained.[24] It is also used to describe the difference between heritability estimates researchers calculate using twin study data versus the usually much lower estimates they calculate based on molecular genetic studies.

Two years prior to the appearance of "missing heritability," I published a book titled *The Missing Gene: Psychiatry, Heredity, and the Fruitless Search for Genes.*[25] My use of the word "missing" in 2006, however, differed from the way that genetic researchers have used it since 2008. I argued that there is little, if any, scientifically acceptable evidence pointing to the existence of predisposing genes for the major psychiatric disorders. For people convinced that family, twin, and adoption studies have provided such evidence—and I will argue in Chapters 3 through 6 that these studies have provided no such evidence—schizophrenia genes are "missing" because researchers haven't yet found them, or because the claimed gene associations or discoveries "explain only a small portion of the variance," or possibly because earlier heritability estimates are too high.

If the critics are right that heritability estimates mislead the public and the research community alike, and that heritability is "one of the most misleading terms in the history of science," this is one aspect of the decades of false-alarm gene discovery claims I discuss below.

Linkage and Candidate Gene Studies

Linkage Studies

English-language schizophrenia molecular genetic study publications first appeared in the 1970s. In a 1973 study, a research group claimed that their "results suggest that there may be genes linked to the *Gc* locus that cause psychosis in general and that there may be genes linked to the *Gm* and/or Rhesus systems that cause schizophrenia."[26]

By the 1960s, there were two main ways that psychiatric genetics and its supporters viewed schizophrenia. Some saw it being caused by a single gene combined with incidental or minor environmental factors, while others saw it as a "polygenic disorder" caused by many genes in combination with environmental triggers. An example of the first approach is seen in a

1964 article by Julian Huxley, Ernst Mayr, Humphry Osmond, and Abram Hoffer, who wrote, "It now appears clear that schizophrenia, at least in the great majority of cases, is based on a single partially dominant gene with low penetrance."[27] The "low penetrance" aspect was needed to account for how schizophrenia showed up in family pedigrees (see Chapter 3) and the fact that schizophrenia concordance among monozygotic (identical) twins was well below 100 percent (see Chapter 5). British psychiatric geneticist Eliot Slater also supported the single-gene approach.[28]

An example of the second approach is seen in a 1967 paper by Irving Gottesman and James Shields. They proposed a *polygenic model* for schizophrenia, which "involves positing a large proportion of cases as being polygenically determined. Thus the disorder would be treated like a threshold character ... whose phenotypic appearance would depend on both the number of genes present and the amount of stress."[29] They believed that schizophrenia environmental factors are "nonspecific and idiosyncratic."[30]

In a *linkage study*, researchers attempt to identify genetic markers associated with a presumed disease gene among consanguineous family members. Findings are often represented as a logarithm of odds (LOD) score, which expresses the probability that the linkage occurred by chance. Linkage studies attempt to identify areas of the chromosome where major relevant genes might be located, but they are unable to identify genes of small effect.

The "Euphoria of the 1980s." A major push to identify genes causing schizophrenia began in the 1980s. A linkage study used to discover the gene causing Huntington's Disease in the early part of that decade gave rise to expectations that investigators would soon discover genes causing the major psychiatric disorders as well.[31]

The linkage era was characterized by what Robert Plomin called in 2013 the "euphoria of the 1980s."[32] Also looking back in 2013, Faraone wrote, "In the 1970s and 1980s, hope ran high as new methods in molecular genetics promised quick discoveries and answers to basic questions of etiology and pathophysiology."[33] Even critics were susceptible to "euphoria of the 1980s" hype. In their important 1984 critical chapter on schizophrenia genetics in *Not in Our Genes: Biology, Ideology, and Human Nature*, Richard Lewontin and colleagues added what appears to be a last-minute footnote acknowledging the "serious research programs now under way in several laboratories to make gene libraries from schizophrenics and isolate and clone the 'schizophrenic genes' with a view to studying their possible replacement."[34]

A widely reported yet non-replicated schizophrenia gene discovery was published in 1988 by the Sherrington/Gurling group, who believed they had found "the first strong evidence for the involvement of a single gene in the causation of schizophrenia."[35] A November 10, 1988, front-page *New York Times* article about this study proclaimed, "*Schizophrenia Study Finds Strong Signs of Hereditary Cause.*"[36] The *Times* also reported subsequently non-replicated schizophrenia gene discoveries in 1995, 1997, 2002, 2006,

2008, and 2013, with headlines such as "*Brain-Tied Gene Defect May Explain Why Schizophrenics Hear Voices,*" "*Schizophrenia May Be Tied To 2 Genes, Research Finds,*" "*Schizophrenia as Misstep by Giant Gene,*" "*Study Ties Genetic Variations to Schizophrenia,*" and "*5 Disorders Share Genetic Risk Factors, Study Finds.*"[37]

As I write these lines, a new schizophrenia gene discovery claim is being widely reported in the media, with a *Washington Post* headline reading, as if five decades of false-alarm schizophrenia gene discovery claims had never happened, "*Researchers Identify New Genetic Link to Schizophrenia.*"[38] Peter Conrad observed that "the news media are a critical vehicle for disseminating new scientific findings into the culture."[39] The media can also be a vehicle for disseminating dubious scientific claims, and then reporting little or nothing when these claims turn out to be false. This captures, in a nutshell, the past four decades of mainstream media "genes for behavior" reporting.

There is no need to go deeper into schizophrenia linkage research because the entire enterprise, as psychiatric geneticists now recognize, produced no replicated findings of causative genes.[40] By 1993 Kendler was describing "the initial strong positive evidence of linkage, followed first by uniformly negative results in all independent studies and then by an inability of the original investigators to replicate their own work."[41]

The Candidate Gene Era in Psychiatry

The period 1990–2010 has been called the "golden age" of behavioral candidate gene studies, but the findings turned out to be fool's gold.[42] A psychiatric *candidate gene association study* attempts to identify genetic influences on a condition by generating hypotheses about it, and then identifying genes that might play a role causing it. Genes become schizophrenia "candidates" based on their role in influencing brain functions believed to be related to the condition. A candidate gene has been defined as "a gene believed a priori to be involved in the pathophysiology of the disorder."[43]

Although many replicated gene associations were claimed in this era, it is now widely recognized that the schizophrenia candidate gene era, like the previous and overlapping linkage era, was a bust. A 2015 review by M. S. Farrell and leading psychiatric genetic researchers such as Lynn DeLisi, Michael O'Donovan, Patrick Sullivan, Pamela Sklar, and Michael Owen listed the main schizophrenia candidate genes that had been put forward for years as possible schizophrenia gene discoveries, such as DISC1, CHRNA7, DRD4, COMT, MTHFR, NRG1, and concluded:

> None of the historical candidate genes can be unequivocally excluded as a genetic risk factor for schizophrenia. However, we can state with high confidence that the large common variant genetic effects originally reported in many initial candidate gene studies are highly unlikely to be true.[44]

The failure of traditional schizophrenia candidate gene studies was confirmed two years later by another group.[45] A similar process occurred in the area of major depression.[46]

Psychologist Stuart Ritchie recalled in 2020 that when he was an undergraduate student between 2005 and 2009, "candidate gene studies were the subject of intense and excited discussion. By the time I got my PhD in early 2014, they were almost entirely discredited."[47] For Ritchie, who otherwise strongly supports behavioral genetic research and theories, "reading through the candidate gene literature is, in hindsight, a surreal experience: they were building a massive edifice of detailed studies on foundations that we now know to be completely false."[48]

How Failure Happened

Flint, Greenspan, and Kendler attempted to come to grips with the reality that "literally thousands of papers reporting the results of physiological candidate gene association tests. ... are now considered to be false positives." This led to their 2020 conclusion that "it's not too harsh to say simply that these studies have taught us nothing useful about the genetic basis of psychiatric disease."[49]

The first reason candidate gene studies failed, according to Flint and colleagues, was the difficulty of picking a good candidate gene. The second reason was "poor analysis." The third reason was that case and control groups were not "equivalent in all respects other than the disease being tested." The fourth reason was that "it made such a good story; it just had to be true."[50]

An additional reason relates directly to the replication crisis I discussed in Chapter 1. By Plomin's 2018 tally, for schizophrenia alone, "over 1,000 papers reported candidate gene results for more than 700 genes." Plomin then asked, "how can so many published papers have got it so wrong?" One reason he gave was "chased P values."[51] This refers to researchers using their hidden flexibility in non-preregistered studies to produce statistically significant "gene-associations" when none existed in reality. In other words, p-hacking seems to have played a role in producing false-positive findings. From his 2018 vantage point, Plomin recognized that the candidate gene era was "a flop."[52]

Among the many "surreal" candidate gene era gene discovery claims, we find a 2005 association between two genes and "creative dance performance,"[53] a 2006 claim of a gene association for "loneliness,"[54] a 2008 gene that predicted voter turnout in a U.S. presidential election,[55] a 2010 claim that a particular gene "conferred an increased risk of joining a gang and using a weapon in a fight for males but not for females,"[56] and a 2014 report of a gene "associated with credit card borrowing behavior."[57] Behavioral candidate gene "discoveries" were all the rage. And then they weren't.[58]

Schizophrenia Candidate Gene Discovery False Alarms

It therefore is established that schizophrenia linkage and candidate gene association studies were a failure. The world's leading schizophrenia researchers now recognize this, at the same time claiming that newer GWAS and PRS studies have finally delivered the goods. I will examine these claims later, but for now I will document gene discovery statements by leading psychiatric genetic researchers during the candidate gene era.

The following quotations are found in the 1997–2010 writings of some of the world's leading researchers and authors claiming discoveries or likely discoveries based on schizophrenia linkage and candidate gene studies.

- 1997—**Edward Shorter,** author of *A History of Psychiatry*: "By 1995, the gene or genes causing schizophrenia had been tentatively placed somewhere on chromosome 6."[59]
- 1997—**Ming Tsuang** and **Stephen Faraone:** "In our view, schizophrenia researchers appear to have found genes that exert a small effect on the onset of schizophrenia."[60]
- 2002—**C. Robert Cloninger:** "Research on the genetic basis of mental disorders crossed a major watershed this summer. For the first time, specific genes have been discovered that influence susceptibility to schizophrenia … .The discovery of some of the pathogenic molecular mechanisms associated with schizophrenia is truly a landmark event in the history of psychiatry."[61]
- 2003—**Thomas Insel** and **Francis Collins:** "Finding genetic factors in mental disorders, whether via linkage or association studies, has proven expensive and, until recently, frustrating. In the past year, several promising candidates have emerged as vulnerability genes for schizophrenia, including neuregulin-1, catechol O-methyltransferase, dysbindin, and G72."[62]
- 2004—**Amanda Elkin, Sridevi Kalidindi,** and **Peter McGuffin:** "Schizophrenia genes have been found at last."[63]
- 2005—**A. H. Fanous** and **Kenneth Kendler:** "Despite years of pessimism, the first generation of linkage and association studies in schizophrenia has succeeded in identifying replicated susceptibility genes."[64]
- 2005—**Paul Harrison** and **Daniel Weinberger:** "A way forward is provided by the recent identification of several putative [schizophrenia] susceptibility genes (including neuregulin, dysbindin, COMT, DISC1, RGS4, GRM3, and G72) … .The evidence for several of the genes is now strong."[65]
- 2005—**Patrick Sullivan:** "Despite the limitations of the accumulated linkage and association studies, there are good suggestions that these studies have identified plausible candidate genes for schizophrenia."[66]
- 2010—**Jonathan Flint, Ralph Greenspan,** and **Kendler:** "While this does not mean that all these regions [of the genome] will yield genes

[for schizophrenia] (some could still be false positives), it is likely that at least some of them may do so."[67]

Commenting on such statements, psychiatric researcher Timothy Crow wrote in 2008 that although the "schizophrenia gene pond" was "empty," this "chorus of reviews ... pervades the literature and will convince all but the most inquisitive that a solid foundation of evidence supports the pathophysiological relevance of these candidate genes."[68] When we evaluate *current* claims of replicated gene associations or discoveries by the world's top researchers, we must remember that many of them were saying these things in an era they *now* recognize to have been a "flop." This was one aspect of my evaluation of Plomin's 2018 book *Blueprint: How DNA Makes Us Who We Are*, and we should keep in mind Crow's "chorus of reviews" comment when attempting to understand later claims based on newer methods—same chorus, different lyrics.[69]

Critics in the Candidate Gene Era were Right

At a time when some of the world's leading psychiatric genetic researchers were claiming replicated gene associations and discoveries for schizophrenia and other major psychiatric disorders (although others were urging more caution), I published books in 2004 and 2006 where I argued that these studies were in fact producing false-positive *non*-findings.[70] I published a subsequent article on the topic in 2012.[71] In *The Missing Gene*, I concluded that psychiatry and psychiatric genetics had failed to discover genes that predispose for psychiatric conditions, and that "genes for the major mental disorders are unlikely to exist."[72] Looking back from the current vantage point, most genetic researchers would probably acknowledge that I was right in saying, in 2006, that schizophrenia molecular genetic research had produced nothing other than false alarms, and that the 2006 "schizophrenia gene pond" was indeed empty.

Kenneth Kendler and I had an exchange in a 2005 edition of the *American Journal of Psychiatry*, that is, in the heyday of the candidate gene era and before the publication of the first schizophrenia GWAS. In response to a previous Kendler article, I wrote that purely environmental theories of schizophrenia predict "(1) familial clustering, (2) a higher concordance of identical versus fraternal twins [see Chapter 4], and (3) a failure to find genes, and this is what we find."[73] In his 2005 response, Kendler wrote,

Dr. Joseph argues that current efforts at gene finding for psychiatric disorders have been unsuccessful. Although there certainly have been problems with replication, I disagree with his interpretation. For example, a recent well-done meta-analysis of schizophrenia linkage studies identified a number of genomic regions with substantial cross-study agreement. Several susceptibility genes for schizophrenia are beginning to be replicated at rates that are hard to explain if the original findings were false positive. I recently summarized this evidence for [the] dysbindin [candidate gene] in the *Journal*, and since then, two further positive reports have been published.[74]

Kendler was referring to a 2004 article where he concluded that, based on *dysbindin* candidate gene findings, "perhaps a corner has been turned in our long struggle."[75] A corner was turned, but it led straight to the schizophrenia "gene graveyard" that 12 years earlier, another leading researcher had feared could become the ultimate resting place of schizophrenia molecular genetic research.[76]

History shows that I was right in 2005 and that one of the world's leading psychiatric genetic researchers was wrong. In the same year, we saw that Fanous and Kendler wrote, "Despite years of pessimism, the first generation of linkage and association studies in schizophrenia has succeeded in identifying replicated susceptibility genes." A year later, I responded to Fanous and Kendler, "I disagree, and it is likely that these claims will share the same fate as other such unsubstantiated claims we have seen over the past decades."[77] Right again, and psychiatrist Steve Pittelli was also right, as seen in a 2003 letter he published in the same top journal.[78] A few years later, Pittelli submitted a letter to another psychiatric journal where he questioned a different gene discovery claim. The editors wrote back, saying they would consider printing his letter only if he could get two other psychiatrists to vouch for his character.[79]

Toward a "Null Field" of Science?

In my 2012 article, I wrote that the probable outcome of psychiatric molecular genetic research would be that genes will not be found because they do not exist, and that psychiatric genetics eventually would be recognized as a "null field" of science. As professor of epidemiology and population health John Ioannidis defined it, a *null field* is an area of research "with absolutely no yield of true scientific information … .The extent that observed findings deviate from what is expected by chance alone would be simply a pure measure of the prevailing bias."[80] For example, even if its top researchers are showered with hundreds of millions of dollars in research grant funding and awards, a field dedicated to studying how differing parenting methods cause Huntington's Disease will eventually become a null field.

The authors of the 2015 Farrell et al. review article argued that while the candidate gene approach in psychiatry was a failure, it helped set the stage for GWAS "successes."[81] Here we see a parallel between psychiatric genetics and companies producing and selling psychotropic drugs. Drug companies recognize how bad their previous (now generic) drugs were when promoting expensive new patented drugs. Psychiatric molecular genetic researchers recognize how bad their previous methods were when promoting new gene-discovery methods. In both cases, it's more about marketing and brand promotion than it is about science.

Sociologists Examine Psychiatric Genetics and "Complexity"

In 2019, sociologists Michael Arribas-Ayllon, Andrew Bartlett, and Jamie Lewis published *Psychiatric Genetics: From Hereditary Madness to Big Biology*.[82] The authors were outsiders to psychiatric genetics, although they spent time in the field's UK facilities. In reference to my 2012 article, Arribas-Ayllon and colleagues recognized that psychiatric genetics was indeed approaching null field status around their first contact with the field in 2008–2010, only to be "saved" by what they saw as positive gene associations produced by GWAS studies using large samples produced by gene-finding consortiums I will soon discuss.[83]

Schizophrenia genetic researchers can always explain failure by pointing to the supposed "complexity" of the condition. In 1991, Neil Risch expressed the view that psychiatric disorders are "diseases" that have "complex, mysterious etiologies."[84] Not only do such statements help explain failure, they also help portray the causes of schizophrenia, psychosis, depression, anxiety, and psychiatric conditions in general as so mysterious and difficult to understand that only experts in psychiatry, genetics, and other fields can attempt to get a handle on them.

Arribas-Ayllon and colleagues saw complexity in psychiatric genetics as a rhetorical device that provides "a means to rescue research programmes from the failures of the past."[85] It allows researchers to switch focus from previous failed attempts to identify genes of large effect to subsequent attempts to identify many genes of small effect. "The emerging view of complexity," they wrote, "is one that attributes increasing significance to polygenetic, multifactorial causation, distancing the field from a simple Mendelian mode of inheritance. Complexity becomes a constitutive part of the phenomena being studied."[86]

In the next section, I will explore the question of whether psychiatric genetics was really "saved" by GWAS and PRS studies.

The Genome-Wide Association Study and Polygenic Risk Score Era

Genome-wide Association Studies

"If 2010 was a precarious time for psychiatric GWAS," Arribas-Ayllon and colleagues wrote, "by 2012, the further growth of consortium-based GWAS had meant that psychiatric genetics had escaped the null field."[87] But is this really the case?

Since the completion of the Human Genome Project in the early 2000s, psychiatry and other behavioral fields have placed hope on *genome-wide association studies* (commonly known as "GWAS," pronounced "GEE-wahs"). These supposedly "hypothesis-free" studies use modern gene sequencing technology, which is constantly becoming cheaper, faster, and more fine grained, to rapidly scan markers across the genomes of ever-increasing numbers of affected and non-affected people to find common genetic variants associated with diseases or behaviors. A GWAS attempts to identify SNPs significantly associated with the condition or characteristic under study. The statistical associations between marker SNPs and schizophrenia take advantage of a crucial physical fact of DNA, called linkage disequilibrium (LD) that the closer genes are to each other on a strand of DNA, the more likely they will travel together ("co-segregate"). Thus, SNPs that are "statistically significant" in association with schizophrenia serve as proxies for hypothetical deviant schizophrenogenic genes nearby.

However, as GWAS pioneer Jonathan Flint and colleagues repeatedly stressed, "A GWAS does not find association with a gene." A GWAS finds associations with a locus, which

> is a geneticist's term for place—a place in the genome where the genetic variant is found ... .If the variant is found by a GWAS altered a coding region, as was initially hoped, then it would be straightforward to say which genes were involved in the trait under investigation. But GWAS hits turned out *not* to be coding for SNPs.[88]

Because multiple comparisons are made, the GWAS significance threshold is very high, usually 5×10^{-8}. To repeat: a GWAS does not identify actual causative genes.

The Psychiatric Genetics Consortium

The GWAS era began around 2005. Two years later, the Wellcome Trust GWAS was published, which looked at common medical conditions and one psychiatric diagnosis (bipolar disorder).[89] In the same year, psychiatric genetic researchers from around the world formed the Psychiatric Genetics Consortium (PGC) to pool resources and expand sample sizes. According to its website, the PGC "is one of the largest and most innovative and productive experiments in the history of psychiatry. The central idea of the PGC is [to] leverage global collaboration to advance genetic discovery of biologically, clinically, and therapeutically meaningful insights."[90] As of February 2022, the PGC had "800+ investigators from 36 countries and >400K subjects. The PGC has attracted a cadre of outstanding scientists whose careers center on our work."[91] The PGC is funded largely by the U.S. National Institute for Mental Health (NIMH),[92] and was formed on the basis of researchers' and institutions' willingness to share raw data and expertise in order to obtain large-enough samples to produce discoveries.

The PGC has several workgroups for specific conditions. For our purposes, of interest is the Schizophrenia Working Group. This group has been a component of the PGC since 2007, and its membership has grown to include over 500 investigators from more than 100 institutions representing around 45 countries.[93] A center of research is the Stanley Center for Psychiatric Research at the Broad Institute, located in Boston, Massachusetts. In 2014, the Stanley Center received a $650 million funding commitment from a wealthy donor to help in the search for genes.[94] According to its website,

> The mission of the Stanley Center for Psychiatric Research at Broad Institute is to reduce the burden of serious mental illness through research. The increasingly successful discovery of genetic variants associated with disease is only the beginning. Our goal is not to end with a list of genes, but to contribute to new understandings of pathogenesis, the identification of biomarkers, and above all, new treatments.[95]

I now briefly describe selected PGC studies that have been published since 2013.

2013 "Cross Disorder Group" study

In 2013 there appeared a well-publicized report from the "Cross Disorder Group" of the PGC, whose authors claimed to have identified shared genes associated with five psychiatric disorders: autism spectrum disorder, attention/deficit-hyperactivity disorder (ADHD), bipolar disorder, major depressive disorder, and schizophrenia.[96]

2014 Schizophrenia GWAS

A 2014 study by the Schizophrenia Working Group, based on 36,989 people diagnosed with schizophrenia (cases) and 113,075 controls, identified 108 regions (loci) of the genome said to be associated with schizophrenia.[97] The study was based on the researchers' belief that "schizophrenia is a highly heritable disorder," and the reported findings included the identification of "128 independent associations spanning 108 conservatively defined loci that meet genome-wide significance, 83 of which have not been previously reported."[98] According to the researchers, variation on the schizophrenia liability scale explained by genome-wide significant loci was only 3.4 percent.[99]

This study played a big role in supporting the idea that a GWAS based on large samples obtained through international cooperation could identify genomic regions harboring schizophrenia genes. The study's "Competing Interests" statement read in part, "Several of the authors are employees of the following pharmaceutical companies; Pfizer … F. Hoffman-La Roche … Eli Lilly … and Janssen." Most of the other researchers declared no competing interests.[100]

The 2016 "Synaptic pruning" study

Another publicized gene discovery claim was the *C4* variant "synaptic pruning" study published by Sekar and colleagues in 2016.[101] As described in an article about this study, Sekar at al. reported "that variation in the configuration of *C4* alleles alters gene expression among individuals, and genotypes that increase *C4* expression are associated with higher risk of developing schizophrenia."[102] The authors declared no competing financial interests.

2022 Schizophrenia GWAS

The 2022 Schizophrenia Working Group GWAS publication was based on more than doubling the 2014 sample to 76,755 people diagnosed with schizophrenia (cases) and 243,649 controls. The researchers now reported "common variant associations at 287 distinct genomic loci." Using fine-mapping and functional genomic data, they identified "120 genes (106 protein-coding) that are likely to underpin associations at some of these loci, including 16 genes with credible causal non-synonymous or untranslated region variation."[103]

According to the researchers, variation on the schizophrenia liability scale explained by genome-wide significant loci was only 2.4 percent, which despite doubling the sample size was lower than the 2014 result, that is, 3.4 percent.[104] The modest 2.4 percent "variation explained by" calculation was reported in the body of the article but was not elaborated upon, and it was not mentioned in the abstract. The study's lengthy "Competing Interests" section showed that many of the researchers taking part in this project had financial ties to the drug companies.

Criticism of Schizophrenia GWAS Research

Schizophrenia GWAS research has been criticized on several grounds. To begin, we saw in Chapter 1 that the reliability and validity of a schizophrenia diagnosis are questionable. Schizophrenia is not diagnosed by medical tests but instead by vaguely defined behaviors, where different people can display different sets of behaviors (symptoms). For this reason alone, all research based on a diagnosis of "schizophrenia" begins on shaky ground. If schizophrenia is not a valid concept, and if it cannot be reliably identified, molecular genetic studies of "schizophrenia" will produce spurious results in part because researchers may be studying the genes of many people who do not really "have" schizophrenia.

We have seen that a schizophrenia GWAS identifies regions of the genome ("hits") "associated with" the condition. It does not identify genes that cause it, and "associated with" does not mean "caused by." The classic example is that if red-haired people in a given society are persecuted, and for this reason alone many red-haired people suffer from depression, it doesn't mean that genes for red hair cause depression. This finding would indicate only that genes for red hair are *associated with* depression, not that they *cause* depression.

The general critique of GWAS involves other areas such as population stratification, questionable assumptions, questionable research practices (QRPs), and conflicts of interest.

Population Stratification

A potential GWAS confounding factor is *population stratification* (PS), which refers to differences in allele frequencies between cases and controls due to systematic differences in ancestry, rather than to the association of disease with genes. In gene-association studies

> population stratification is a primary consideration in studies of the genetic determinants of human traits. Failure to control for it may lead to confounding, causing a study to fail for lack of significant results or resources to be wasted following false positive signals.[105]

Although researchers claim they are able to control for PS, others disagree. A *confound* is an unforeseen or uncontrolled-for factor that threatens the validity of conclusions researchers draw from their studies. Confounding occurs when the association between two variables is caused by a third variable that influences both, and is also relevant to the twin and adoption studies I will explore in the chapters to follow.

In a 2021 analysis, behavioral genetics critic Evan Charney described the potentially confounding influence of population stratification:

> Structured populations, which are most populations, are considered an omnipresent threat to the validity of genetic association studies due to population stratification. Population stratification arises when differences in allele frequencies between cases and controls, ascribed to genetic risk factors, are actually due to ancestry related population genetic differences.[106]

Indeed, when such differences in allele frequencies between cases and controls correlate with differences in environmental influences between cases and controls, GWAS researchers might erroneously attribute the effects of these environmental influences to genetics.

Charney concluded that the methods genetic researchers use to effectively deal with the PS problem are inadequate. In a 2022 article, biologists Graham Coop and Molly Przeworski wrote that potential biases introduced by population stratification "highlight a central challenge to identifying genetic causes of behavioral traits, the immense difficulty of disentangling population stratification from biological and social effects."[107]

In relation to potential PS confounds in a GWAS or a PRS, Ken Richardson and Mike Jones concluded that in studies of cognitive ability and educational attainment, "genetic variation ... covaries with social class."[108] This finding is relevant to schizophrenia, where the working class and the poor are disproportionally diagnosed with the condition.[109]

The potentially confounding influence of population stratification is a major problem in GWAS research, and may have contributed to producing results similar to the spurious results produced by the earlier linkage and candidate gene studies.

Questionable Assumptions

Schizophrenia GWAS researchers assume that heritability is a useful and important concept, and that schizophrenia heritability is roughly 80 percent. We saw that a major criticism of heritability estimates is that researchers who use them must assume that genes and environment do not interact, when clearly they do. If the critics are right that heritability estimates are misleading and are based on questionable or false assumptions, including the questionable or false assumptions in twin research I will examine in Chapters 4 and 5, this by itself would throw a monkey wrench into GWAS calculations, and lead to the decades of false-alarms we have witnessed.

Questionable Research Practices

In 2016, behavioral geneticist Eric Turkheimer wrote that "genome-wide association is unapologetic, high-tech p-hacking."[110] In a subsequent 2019 blogpost titled "P-hacking in GWAS," he elaborated that although "unapologetic p-hacking is way better than secretive p-hacking," it is still p-hacking. "GWAS methods are public and open," Turkheimer wrote, "but that doesn't mean they are scientifically desirable." GWAS "significance testing" puts a "scientific gloss on a process that consists essentially of printing out a big table of correlation coefficients and circling the [significant] ones..."[111]

By definition, a scientific fishing expedition is a hypothesis-free method, where researchers base their conclusions on significant associations that in the GWAS context pop up on a Manhattan plot. As the author of an article about QRPs in psychiatric research wrote,

> The term *fishing expedition* is used to describe what researchers do when they indiscriminately examine associations between different combinations of variables not with the intention of testing a priori hypotheses but with the hope of finding something that is statistically significant in the data.[112]

It could be argued that a GWAS is a type of scientific fishing expedition.

Increasing the Sample Size and Potential Conflicts of Interest

In 2021, behavioral geneticist K. Paige Harden recalled listening to many scientific talks prior to 2013 about efforts to find genes associated with various life outcomes. "All of these ended pretty much the same way" she wrote, "We haven't found anything *yet*, but just wait until we get more people!"[113]

In his 2012 "Don't Give Up on GWAS" article, PGC leader Patrick Sullivan urged "major funding sources worldwide" to keep on funding because the "outcomes of GWAS cannot be declared until sample sizes are sufficiently large. If samples are sufficient, GWAS can deliver fundamental knowledge about genetic architecture, identify specific loci for biological follow-up and localize pathways altered in disease."[114] On the other hand, as Turkheimer wrote in his 2019 blogpost in a general comment, "increasing [a GWAS] sample size endlessly until some unpredicted correlation reaches an arbitrary level of significance, sounds a lot like p-hacking to me."[115]

Although he declared no conflict of interest in 2012, in a 2018 article Sullivan's "conflict of interest" statement read, "PFS is a scientific advisor for Pfizer and Lundbeck and received an honorarium from F. Hoffmann-La Roche AG." The statement also recognized that "multiple drug companies work with the PGC in a manner equivalent to academic investigators."[116]

There is a symbiotic relationship between psychiatry, psychiatric genetics, and the companies that produce and sell psychiatric drugs. All have a vital and mutual interest in convincing the public that psychiatric conditions are real diseases, in need of medication like other diseases.[117] They often say that people diagnosed with schizophrenia need medication in the same way as people diagnosed with diabetes mellitus need insulin. The drugs prescribed to people diagnosed with schizophrenia are profitable and are sometimes prescribed for a lifetime. Companies and researchers believe they will be able to design and patent drugs targeted at a person's genotype, and that they stand to profit even more in the future.

Former Editor-in-Chief of *The New England Journal of Medicine* Marcia Angell wrote in 2000 about the potentially corrupting relationship between "academic medicine" and industry:

The ties between clinical researchers and industry include not only grant support, but also a host of other financial arrangements. Researchers serve as consultants to companies whose products they are studying, join advisory boards and speakers' bureaus, enter into patent and royalty arrangements, agree to be the listed authors of articles ghostwritten by interested companies, promote drugs and devices at company sponsored symposiums, and allow themselves to be plied with expensive gifts and trips to luxurious settings. Many also have equity interest in the companies.[118]

Statements listing researchers' "competing interests" in molecular genetic research publications are a positive development, even though these statements fail to disclose how much various researchers are paid by the drug companies ($1, $1,000, $1,000,000?). Consumers of psychiatric research should be supplied with this information, since financial conflicts of interest can influence how researchers perform their studies and interpret their data. In addition, to ensure maximum visibility, competing interest statements should be placed at the end of an article's abstract. Other ways researchers believe the product potentially could be monetized, from which they could reap financial rewards, are through the marketing of direct-to-consumer genetic tests such as 23&Me, and through companies selling products aimed at marital partners and post-conception embryo selection.

Other GWAS Claims

I have already listed some unlikely and even humorous "findings" from the candidate gene era. The GWAS method has produced some of its own. The authors of various GWAS publications claimed to have found significant loci for behavioral characteristics that include getting concussions[119]; self-reported childhood maltreatment[120]; crying habits[121]; female sexual dysfunction[122]; food liking[123]; household income[124]; ice cream flavor preferences[125]; leadership traits[126]; loneliness[127]; being a morning person[128]; musical beat synchronization[129]; risk taking behavior[130]; regular attendance at a sports club, pub, or religious group[131]; sexual behavior[132]; television watching[133]; and "white wine liking."[134] These supposed findings are a huge red flag for potentially spurious results in schizophrenia GWAS investigations, just as they were during the candidate gene era.

Polygenic Risk Score Studies

In *Blueprint*, Plomin championed the relatively new *polygenic risk score* (PRS) method as a "new fortune-telling device" that uses a person's genetic profile to "predict psychological traits like depression, schizophrenia and school achievement."[135] He described the PRS method as a molecular genetic technique that combines statistically significant and nonsignificant individual SNP associations to produce a polygenic (composite) risk score. Others have described polygenic risk scores as "generally constructed as weighted sum scores of risk alleles using effect sizes from genome-wide association studies as their weights."[136] Polygenic risk scores are also known as genetic risk scores, genomic risk profile scores, and polygenic scores. They are expressed as a percentage.

The PRS practice of combining statistically significant and non-significant SNPs assumes that all play some role in causing variation in the trait/condition in question. According to Flint and colleagues, schizophrenia polygenic scores "exploit the fact that many variants failing to meet genome-wide significance could still have an effect on the trait." (If something only *could* be true, it is not a "fact.") They believe that if "schizophrenia has a polygenic basis of inheritance, that is, that there are many loci, perhaps thousands, each of small effect contributing to disease risk…then the effect of variants in one population (or group of patients) should predict disease in another."[137]

Criticism of PRS

Most problems that apply to GWAS apply to polygenic risk scores as well, which are derived from GWAS results. Among these problems are the questionable validity and reliability of a schizophrenia diagnosis, non-causative correlations, environmental confounds such as population stratification, boosting sample sizes to find significant results and other QRPs, genetic confirmation bias, and potential conflicts of interest. A 2022 study discussed the "low portability of polygenic scores (PGSs) across global populations," and found a "dramatic reduction in portability of PGSs trained using Northwestern European individuals and applied to nine ancestry groups."[138] If polygenic scores measure disease risk as opposed to population characteristics, we would expect scores to validate across population groups in the same way as most medical tests do.

Like GWAS results, a polygenic risk score reflects correlational data and does not identify genes that play a role in causing behavioral differences or psychiatric conditions. In the words of historian of science Nathaniel Comfort,

> A polygenic score is a correlation coefficient. A GWAS identifies single nucleotide polymorphisms (SNPs) in the DNA that correlate with the trait of interest. The SNPs are markers only. Although they might, in some cases, suggest genomic neighbourhoods in which to search for genes that directly affect the trait, the polygenic score itself is in no sense causal.[139]

Because Plomin strongly advocated for the polygenic risk score method in *Blueprint*, in Turkheimer's view Plomin abandoned "the original task of figuring out which gene does what on a biological level," because, as correlational data, "polygenic scores achieve their predictive power by abdicating any claim to biological meaning. SNPs are summed willy-nilly across chromosomes."[140] In an interview, veteran psychiatric genetic researcher Elliot Gershon described PRS as "sort of a mindless score," and that "you can't really tell anything from the polygenic risk factor."[141] Sociologist/criminologist Callie Burt described several potential PRS environmental confounds and concluded that scores should be used "sparingly and cautiously with caveats placed front and center."[142] Medical researcher Keith Baverstock called polygenic risk scores "a dangerous delusion."[143]

In *Blueprint*, Plomin called for ending the idea that specific behavioral or psychiatric conditions exist, arguing that they are caused not by genes specific to each condition, but are instead influenced by "generalist genes" falling into "three broad genetic clusters." This means that we will have to "tear up our diagnostic manuals based on symptoms."[144] Plomin predicted the "demise" of psychiatric conditions, since "there are no disorders to diagnose and there are no disorders to cure."[145] In the same book, he cited research claiming that schizophrenia and other psychiatric conditions are "under substantial genetic influence" and can be predicted by polygenic risk scores.[146] Plomin failed to explain how psychiatric conditions can be studied, predicted, and "substantially genetically influenced" if they do not exist.

Plomin offered several explanations in *Blueprint* for why some of *his own* polygenic risk scores did not match his reality. For example, Plomin's schizophrenia score was in the 85th percentile, even though "I don't feel at all schizophrenic, in the sense of having disorganized thoughts, hallucinations, delusions or paranoia."[147] Rather than offer this result as evidence that polygenic risk scores cannot be trusted—as he easily could have—he seemed to suggest that his high score could be explained by creative thinking and genius. "A nicer way of thinking about my higher than average polygenic risk score for schizophrenia," Plomin wrote, "is to contemplate possible aspects of what at the extreme is called schizophrenia. The best example is a possible link between schizophrenia and creative thinking. Aristotle said, 'no great genius was without a mixture of insanity.'"[148] Genetic confirmation bias can take people to some really unusual places.

What appears to matter most to Plomin now are "DNA fortune-telling" polygenic risk scores and his belief that researchers have found genetic "gold dust, not nuggets. Each speck of gold was not worth much, but scooping up handfuls of gold dust made it possible to predict genetic propensities of individuals."[149] It is probable that Plomin's "gold dust specks" are just the latest version of the genes-for-behavior fool's gold that molecular genetic researchers—misled by twin studies, adoption studies, and heritability estimates—have been collecting for the past half century or so.

Most likely, the polygenic risk score method will become the latest in a long line of failed molecular genetic methods in the area of human behavior, whose failures are usually only recognized after the latest-and-greatest method is said to have finally revealed the long-lost "genes for behavior." In his 2014 book *Misbehaving Science: Controversy and the Development of Behavior Genetics*, sociologist Aaron Panofsky described the behavioral genetic gene-discovery failure "coping strategy" of "technological optimism." By this he meant the "optimism that the next level of technology will overcome past disappointments."[150]

Current excitement about PRS in psychiatric genetics and behavioral genetics is likely to fade when it becomes yet another "next level" method that failed. A 2022 PRS study of the supposedly "highly heritable" trait of "educational attainment" (EA), which was based on genetic samples from 3 million individuals, returned results disappointing for behavioral geneticists and their supporters.[151] Kendler and colleagues interpreted the results of this study as evidence that "genetic associations with EA and its health benefits may be mostly indirect."[152] As seen in the example of red hair color leading to depression, an "indirect genetic effect" is another name for an environmental effect.

In my 2015 book *The Trouble with Twin Studies*, I addressed the then-latest-and-greatest molecular genetic method designed to solve the missing heritability problem, called "genome-wide complex trait analysis," or GCTA. Evan Charney described several potential biases in these studies, and concluded that the GCTA search for thousands of genetic variants of tiny effect "is the last gasp of a failed paradigm."[153] I added in 2015 that "although the GCTA approach does appear to be a 'gasp of a failed paradigm,' it is probably not the last gasp."[154] We don't hear much about GCTA these days, but we continue to hear a lot about the "fortune-telling" PRS method in behavioral research.

Assuming that the PRS method will fade into obscurity, like GCTA it will not be the "last gasp of a failed paradigm" for the simple reason that the genetic paradigm is needed by people, institutions, and corporations that profit from it, and by politicians seeking "scientific" justification for preserving the political status quo, which means doing little to improve the abysmal living conditions experienced by so many of the world's people. For all these groups, at least for now, the genetic paradigm is too big to fail.

In the 1850s, a mental disorder called "Drapetomania" was invented by American physician Samuel Cartwright to pathologize people of African descent who tried to escape slavery.[155] There is little doubt that if GWAS and PRS technology had existed during the U.S. Civil War, slave-trading companies and a "Confederate Institute of Mental Health" would have financed them, and Drapetomania GWAS "hits" and polygenic scores would have been published in a "Confederate Journal of Psychiatry."

Most likely, Stuart Ritchie's evaluation of the candidate gene era will be the future consensus evaluation of the schizophrenia GWAS/PRS era as well: "They were building a massive edifice of detailed studies on foundations that we now know to be completely false."

Summary and Conclusions

This chapter began with a brief overview of schizophrenia molecular genetic research. I showed that the practice of estimating heritability is faulty. I then explored the three main (and sometimes overlapping) eras of schizophrenia molecular genetic research: the linkage, candidate gene, and genome-wide association/polygenic risk score eras, followed by a critique of these methods. Despite countless gene discovery claims in the media and in academic works since the 1970s, genes shown to cause schizophrenia and psychosis have not been found. If such genes do not exist, of course, molecular genetic research methods will not be able to "find" them.

Gene discovery claims based on recent schizophrenia GWAS and polygenetic risk score studies should be treated with extreme caution. At best, such studies find gene-behavior associations (correlations) without showing that specific genes play a role in causing schizophrenia and psychosis. Like the older methods, these more recent studies suffer from systematic bias and error, and a reliance on the validity of heritability estimates.

Every media report on new schizophrenia gene-association claims should begin something like this: After 50 years of sometimes sensationalized schizophrenia "gene-association" claims that fell by the wayside, a new claim has appeared. We report on it here, but due to this dreadful track record we advise our readers to treat this new claim with skepticism—similar to the "oh no, not again" skepticism Peanuts comic strip character Charlie Brown responded with whenever Lucy van Pelt asked him to kick the football she was holding. Like thousands of previous reports, it is likely that this one is just another spurious non-finding.

Potentially corrupting factors leading to the past failure of psychiatric genetic linkage and candidate gene studies are also at play in the GWAS/PRS era. These factors include highly financed studies expected to produce results, the need to justify grants and salaries, the close relationship between psychiatric research and the drug companies, protecting the legitimacy of the field, the questionable research practices found in non-preregistered studies, and prestigious journals' desire to publish "exciting" positive findings to generate increased interest and revenues. (Who wants to read about failure?) Plus, the ever-present "it made such a good story; it just had to be true" factor. "If you find a magical hammer that, whenever you swing it, rewards you with funding and professional advancement," wrote Marcus Feldman and Jessica Riskin, "you look at your research area and see nothing but nails. Genome-wide association studies are the social sciences' new magical hammer."[156]

The body of family, twin, and adoption research supposedly established the "high heritability of schizophrenia," which justified the molecular genetic research I described in this chapter. In the next four chapters I will show that these studies are characterized by questionable or false assumptions, QRPs, and other methodological issues. I will show that schizophrenia molecular genetic research is built on a foundation of sand, and that this is the likely explanation for the ongoing half-century-long failure to discover genes that cause schizophrenia.

Notes

1 Conrad, P. (2002), Genetics and Behavior in the News: Dilemmas of a Rising Paradigm, in J. Alper et al. (Eds.), *The Double-Edged Helix: Social Implications of Genetics in a Diverse Society* (pp. 58–79), Baltimore: Johns Hopkins University Press.

2 Insel, T. R. (2022), *Healing: Our Path from Mental Illness to Mental Health*, Penguin Publishing Group. Kindle Edition, p. 132.

3 Joseph, J. (in press), A "Blueprint" for Genetic Determinism: An Appraisal of Robert Plomin's Blueprint: How DNA Makes Us Who We Are, *American Journal of Psychology*.

4 Faraone, S. V., Tsuang, M. T., & Tsuang, D. W. (1999), *Genetics of Mental Disorders*, New York: Guilford, p. 198.

5 Merikangas, K. R., & Risch, N. (2003), Will the Genomics Revolution Revolutionize Psychiatry?, *American Journal of Psychiatry*, 160, 625–635, p. 626. https://doi.org/10.1176/appi.ajp.160.4.625

6 American Psychiatric Association (2013, May 3rd), Chair of DSM-5 Task Force Discusses Future of Mental Health Research; Statement by David Kupfer, M.D., *American Psychiatric Association* [Press release]. https://www.madinamerica.com/wp-content/uploads/2013/05/Statement-from-dsm-chair-david-kupfer-md.pdf

7 Moore, D. S. (2015), *The Developing Genome: An Introduction to Developmental Epigenetics*, New York: Oxford University Press.

8 Charney et al. (2002), Neuroscience Research Agenda to Guide Development of a Pathophysiologically Based Classification System, in Kupfer et al. (Eds.), *A Research Agenda for DSM-V* (pp. 31–83), Washington, DC: American Psychiatric Association, p. 71.

9 Joseph, J. (2015), *The Trouble with Twin Studies: A Reassessment of Twin Research in the Social and Behavioral Sciences*, New York: Routledge, Chapter 8; American Psychiatric Association, 2013, May 3.

10 Faraone, S. V. (2013), Real Progress in Molecular Psychiatric Genetics, *Journal of the American Academy of Child and Adolescent Psychiatry*, 52, 1006–1008. https://doi.org/10.1016/j.jaac.2013.07.014, p. 1007.

11 Faraone et al. (2008), The New Neuropsychiatric Genetics, *American Journal of Medical Genetics Part B (Neuropsychiatric Genetics)* 147B, 1–2, p. 1. https://doi.org/10.1002/ajmg.b.30691

12 Merikangas et al. (2022), What Genes are Differentially Expressed in Individuals with Schizophrenia? A Systematic Review, *Molecular Psychiatry*, 10.1038/s41380-021-01420-7. Advance online publication. https://doi.org/10.1038/s41380-021-01420-7

13 Akingbuwa et al. (2022), Ultra-rare and Common Genetic Variant Analysis Converge to Implicate Negative Selection and Neuronal Processes in the Aetiology of Schizophrenia, *Molecular Psychiatry*, p. 2. Advance online publication, https://doi.org/10.1038/s41380-022-01621-8

14 Flint, J., Greenspan, R. J., & Kendler, K. S. (2020), *How Genes Influence Behavior* (2nd ed.), Oxford, UK: Oxford University Press, p. 98.

15 Hirsch, J. (1997), Some History of Heredity-vs-Environment, Genetic Inferiority at Harvard (?), and the (Incredible) Bell Curve, *Genetica*, 99, 207–224, p. 220. https://doi.org/10.1007/BF02259524

16 Plomin et al. (2013), *Behavioral Genetics* (6th ed.), New York: Worth Publishers, p. 419.

17 Plomin et al., 2013, p. 87.

18 Gottesman, I. I., & Shields, J. (1967), A Polygenic Theory of Schizophrenia, *Proceedings of the National Academy of Sciences of the United States of America, 58*, 199–205, p. 201. https://doi.org/10.1073/pnas.58.1.199

19 Sullivan, P. F., Kendler, K. S., & Neale, M. C. (2003), Schizophrenia as a Complex Trait: Evidence from a Meta-Analysis of Twin Studies, *Archives of General Psychiatry, 60,* 1187–1192. https://doi.org/10.1001/archpsyc.60.12.1187

20 Feldman, M. W., & Riskin, J. (2022, April 21st), Why Biology is Not Destiny [Review of the Book *The Genetic Lottery: Why DNA Matters for Social Equality*, by K. P. Harden], *The New York Review of Books.* https://www.nybooks.com/articles/2022/04/21/why-biology-is-not-destiny-genetic-lottery-kathryn-harden/

21 Robette, N., Génin, E., & Clerget-Darpoux, F. (2022), Heritability: What's the Point? What Is It Not For? A Human Genetics Perspective, *Genetica.* Advance online publication 1/29/2022. https://doi.org/10.1007/s10709-022-00149-7

22 Moore, D. S., & Shenk, D. (2016), The Heritability Fallacy, *WIREs Cognitive Science,* https://doi.org/10.1002/wcs.1400

23 Maher, B. (2008), The Case of the Missing Heritability, *Nature, 456,* 18–2. https://doi.org/10.1038/456018a; Manolio et al. (2009), Finding the Missing Heritability of Complex Diseases, *Nature, 461,* 747–753. https://doi.org/10.1038/nature08494

24 For the first major mainstream academic publication on the "missing heritability" problem, see Manolio et al., 2009.

25 Joseph, J. (2006), *The Missing Gene: Psychiatry, Heredity, and the Fruitless Search for Genes,* New York: Algora.

26 Elston et al. (1973), Possible Linkage Relationships between Certain Blood Groups and Schizophrenia or Other Psychoses, *Behavior Genetics, 3,* 101–106, p. 105. https://doi.org/10.1007/BF01067650

27 Huxley, J., Mayr, E., Osmond, H., & Hoffer, A. (1964), Schizophrenia as a Genetic Morphism, *Nature, 204,* 220–221, p. 220. https://doi.org/10.1038/204220a0

28 Slater, E. (1958), The Monogenic Theory of Schizophrenia, *Acta Genetica et Statistica Medica,* 8(1), 50–56. https://doi.org/10.1159/000151053; Slater, E., & Cowie, V. (1971), *The Genetics of Mental Disorders,* London: Oxford University Press.

29 Gottesman, I. I., & Shields, J. (1967), A Polygenic Theory of Schizophrenia, *Proceedings of the National Academy of Sciences of the United States of America, 58*, 199–205, p. 204. https://doi.org/10.1073/pnas.58.1.199

30 Gottesman, I. I., & Shields, J. (1972), *Schizophrenia and Genetics: A Twin Study Vantage Point,* New York: Academic Press, p. 301.

31 Gusella et al. (1983), A Polymorphic DNA Marker Genetically Linked to Huntington's Disease, *Nature, 306*(5940), 234–238. https://doi.org/10.1038/306234a0

32 Plomin et al., 2013, p. 240.

33 Faraone, 2013, p. 1006.

34 Lewontin, R. C., Rose, S., & Kamin, L. J. (1984), *Not in Our Genes: Biology, Ideology, and Human Nature,* New York: Pantheon, p. 207.

35 Sherrington et al. (1988), Localization of a Susceptibility Locus for Schizophrenia on Chromosome 5, *Nature, 336,* 164–167, p. 164. https://doi.org/10.1038/336164a0

36 https://www.nytimes.com/1988/11/10/us/schizophrenia-study-finds-strong
-signs-of-hereditary-cause.html?pagewanted=all

37 URLs for supposed schizophrenia gene discoveries as reported over the years
in the *New York Times*. https://www.nytimes.com/1995/10/31/science/gene
-hunters-pursue-elusive-and-complex-traits-of-mind.html?pagewanted=all;
https://www.nytimes.com/1997/01/21/science/brain-tied-gene-defect-may
-explain-why-schizophrenics-hear-voices.html; https://www.nytimes.com/2002
/07/04/us/schizophrenia-may-be-tied-to-2-genes-research-finds.html; https://
www.nytimes.com/2006/04/18/science/schizophrenia-as-misstep-by-giant-gene
.html; https://www.nytimes.com/2008/03/28/science/28gene.html?_r=0; https://
www.nytimes.com/2013/03/01/health/study-finds-genetic-risk-factors-shared
-by-5-psychiatric-disorders.html?_r=0;

38 https://www.washingtonpost.com/health/2022/04/06/schizophrenia-genetic
-link/. The original study was Singh et al. (2022), Rare Coding Variants in Ten
Genes Confer Substantial Risk for Schizophrenia, *Nature*. https://doi.org/10
.1038/s41586-022-04556-w

39 Conrad, 2002, p. 59.

40 Arribas-Ayllon, M., Bartlett, A., & Lewis, J. (2019), *Psychiatric Genetics: From
Hereditary Madness to Big Biology*, London: Routledge; Flint, Greenspan, &
Kendler, 2020.

41 Kendler, K. S., & Diehl, S. R. (1993), The Genetics of Schizophrenia: A Current,
Genetic-Epidemiologic Perspective, *Schizophrenia Bulletin, 19*, 261–285, p.
276. https://doi.org/10.1093/schbul/19.2.261

42 Charney, E. (2021), Is This the "Golden Age" of Behavioral Genetics?, *The
Samuel DuBois Cook Center on Social Equity*, p. 8. https://ssrn.com/abstract
=3747229 or https://doi.org/10.2139/ssrn.3747229

43 Hyman, S. E., & Nestler, E. J. (1993), *The Molecular Foundations of Psychiatry*,
Washington, DC: American Psychiatric Press, p. 209.

44 Farrell et al. (2015), Evaluating Historical Candidate Genes for Schizophrenia,
Molecular Psychiatry, 20, 555–562, p. 560. https://doi.org/10.1038/mp.2015.16

45 Johnson et al. (2017), No Evidence That Schizophrenia Candidate Genes Are
More Associated with Schizophrenia Than Noncandidate Genes, *Biological
Psychiatry, 82*, 702–708. https://doi.org/10.1016/j.biopsych.2017.06.033

46 Border et al. (2019), No Support for Historical Candidate Gene or Candidate
Gene-by-Interaction Hypotheses for Major Depression Across Multiple Large
Samples, *American Journal of Psychiatry, 176*, 376–387. https://doi.org/10
.1176/appi.ajp.2018.18070881

47 Ritchie, S. (2020), *Science Fictions: How Fraud, Bias, Negligence, and Hype
Undermine the Search for Truth*, Henry Holt and Company, p. 140.

48 Ritchie, 2020, p. 141

49 Flint, Greenspan, & Kendler, 2020, p. 60.

50 Flint, Greenspan, & Kendler, 2020, pp. 60–62.

51 Plomin, R. (2018), *Blueprint: How DNA Makes Us Who We Are*, Cambridge,
MA: MIT Press, pp. 222–223.

52 Plomin, 2018, p. 224.

53 Bachner-Melman et al. (2005), *AVPR1a* and *SLC6A4* Gene Polymorphisms Are
Associated with Creative Dance Performance, *PLoS Genetics*. https://doi.org
/10.1371/journal.pgen.0010042

54 Boomsma et al. (2006), Genetic Linkage and Association Analysis for Loneliness
in Dutch Twin and Sibling Pairs Points to a Region on Chromosome 12q23-24,
Behavior Genetics, 36, 137–146. https://doi.org/10.1007/s10519-005-9005-z

55 Fowler, J. H., & Dawes, C. T. (2008), Two Genes Predict Voter Turnout, *Journal
of Politics, 70*, 579–594. https://doi.org/10.1017/S0022381608080638

56 Beaver et al. (2010), Monoamine Oxidase A Genotype is Associated with Gang Membership and Weapon Use, *Comprehensive Psychiatry, 51,* 130–134. https://doi.org/10.1016/j.comppsych.2009.03.010

57 De Neve, J., & Fowler, J. H. (2014), Credit Card Borrowing and the Monoamine Oxidase A (MAOA) Gene, *Journal of Economic Behavior and Organization.* https://doi.org/10.2139/ssrn.1457224

58 Charney, E., & English, W. (2012), Candidate Genes and Political Behavior, *American Political Science Review, 106,* 1–34. https://doi.org/10.1017/S0003055411000554

59 Shorter, E. (1997), *A History of Psychiatry*, New York: Wiley, p. 246.

60 Tsuang, M. T., & Faraone, S. V. (1997), *Schizophrenia: The Facts* (2nd ed.), Oxford: Oxford University Press, pp. 52–53.

61 Cloninger, C. R. (2002), The Discovery of Susceptibility Genes for Mental Disorders, *Proceedings of the National Academy of Sciences, 99,* 13365–13367, pp. 13365, 13367. https://www.pnas.org/content/pnas/99/21/13365.full.pdf

62 Insel, T. R, & Collins, F. S. (2003), Psychiatry in the Genomics Era, *American Journal of Psychiatry, 160,* 616–620, p. 618. https://doi.org/10.1176/appi.ajp.160.4.616

63 Elkin, A., Kalidindi, S., McGuffin, P. (2004), Have Schizophrenia Genes Been Found?, *Current Opinion in Psychiatry, 17,* 107–113, p. 107. https://doi.org/10.1097/00001504-200403000-00007

64 Fanous, A. H., & Kendler, K. S. (2005), Genetic Heterogeneity, Modifier Genes, and Quantitative Phenotypes for Psychiatric Illness: Searching for a Framework, *Molecular Psychiatry, 10,* 6–13, pp. 10–11. https://doi.org/10.1038/sj.mp.4001571

65 Harrison, P. J., & Weinberger, D. R. (2005), Schizophrenia Genes, Gene Expression, and Neuropathology: On the Matter of Their Convergence, *Molecular Psychiatry, 10,* 40–45, p. 40. https://doi.org/10.1038/sj.mp.4001558

66 Sullivan, P. F. (2005), The Genetics of Schizophrenia, *PLoS Medicine* 2(7), e212, 0615–0616. https://doi.org/10.1371/journal.pmed.0020212

67 Flint, J., Greenspan, R. J., & Kendler, K. S. (2010), *How Genes Influence Behavior* (1st ed.), Oxford, UK: Oxford University Press, p. 47.

68 Crow, T. J. (2008), The Emperors of the Schizophrenia Polygene Have No Clothes, *Psychological Medicine, 38,* 1681–1685, p. 1681. https://doi.org/10.1017/S0033291708003395

69 Joseph, in press; Plomin, 2018.

70 Joseph, 2004, 2006.

71 Joseph, J. (2012), The "Missing Heritability" of Psychiatric Disorders: Elusive Genes or Non-Existent Genes?, *Applied Developmental Science, 16,* 65–83. https://doi.org/10.1080/10888691.2012.667343

72 Joseph, 2006, p. 263.

73 Joseph, J. (2005), Research Paradigms of Psychiatric Genetics [Letter to the Editor], *American Journal of Psychiatry, 162,* 1985, p. 1985.

74 Kendler, K. S. (2005), Dr. Kendler Responds, *American Journal of Psychiatry, 162,* 1985–1986, p. 1986.

75 Kendler, K. S. (2004), Schizophrenia Genetics and Dysbindin: A Corner Turned?, *American Journal of Psychiatry, 161,* 1533–1536, p. 1535. https://doi.org/10.1176/appi.ajp.161.9.1533

76 Owen, M. J. (1992), Will Schizophrenia Become a Graveyard for Molecular Geneticists?, *Psychological Medicine, 22,* 289–293, p. 290. https://doi.org/10.1176/appi.ajp.161.9.1533

77 Joseph, 2006, p. 234.

78 Pittelli, S. J. (2003), Genetic Link in Schizophrenia [Letter to the Editor], *American Journal of Psychiatry, 160,* 597.

79 Steve Pittelli, personal communication, 5/6/2022.
80 Ioannidis, J. (2005), Why Most Published Research Findings are False, *PLoS Medicine*, 2, 696–701, p. 700. https://doi.org/10.1371/journal.pmed.0020124
81 Farrell et al., 2015, p. 555.
82 Arribas-Ayllon, Bartlett, & Lewis, 2019.
83 Arribas-Ayllon, Bartlett, & Lewis, 2019, p. 215.
84 Risch, N. (1991), Genetic Linkage Studies in Psychiatry: Theoretical Aspects, in Tsuang et al. (Eds.), *Genetic Issues in Psychosocial Epidemiology* (pp. 71–93), New Brunswick, NJ: Rutgers University Press, p. 90.
85 Arribas-Ayllon, Bartlett, & Lewis, 2019, p. 75.
86 Arribas-Ayllon, Bartlett, & Lewis, 2019, pp. 79–80.
87 Arribas-Ayllon, Bartlett, & Lewis, 2019, p. 203.
88 Flint, Greenspan, & Kendler, 2020, p. 79.
89 Wellcome Trust Case Control Consortium (2007), Genome-wide Association Study of 14,000 Cases of Seven Common Diseases and 3,000 Shared Controls, *Nature, 447*, 661–678. https://doi.org/10.1038/nature05911; Klein et al. (2005), Complement Factor H Polymorphism in Age-related Macular Degeneration, *Science, 308*, 5720, 385–389. https://doi.org/10.1126/science.1109557
90 https://www.med.unc.edu/pgc/
91 https://www.med.unc.edu/pgc/about-us/
92 https://www.med.unc.edu/pgc/pgc-workgroups/schizophrenia/
93 https://www.med.unc.edu/pgc/pgc-workgroups/schizophrenia/
94 https://www.broadinstitute.org/news/650-million-commitment-stanley-center -broad-institute-aims-galvanize-mental-illness-research
95 https://www.broadinstitute.org/stanley
96 Cross-Disorder Group of the Psychiatric Genomics Consortium (2013), Identification of Risk Loci with Shared Effects on Five Major Psychiatric Disorders: A Genome-Wide Analysis, *Lancet, 381*, 1371–1379. https://doi.org /10.1016/S0140-6736(12)62129-1
97 Schizophrenia Working Group of the Psychiatric Genomics Consortium (2014), Biological Insights from 108 Schizophrenia-Associated Genetic Loci, *Nature, 511*, 421–427. https://doi.org/10.1038/nature13595
98 Schizophrenia Working Group of the Psychiatric Genomics Consortium, 2014, p. 421. https://doi.org/10.1038/nature13595
99 Schizophrenia Working Group of the Psychiatric Genomics Consortium, 2014, p. 424.
100 Schizophrenia Working Group of the Psychiatric Genomics Consortium, 2014, online version. https://www.nature.com/articles/nature13595
101 Sekar et al. (2016), Schizophrenia Risk from Complex Variation of Complement Component 4, *Nature, 530*, 177–183. https://doi.org/10.1038/nature16549
102 https://www.science.org/doi/10.1126/scitranslmed.aaf3851
103 Schizophrenia Working Group of the Psychiatric Genomics Consortium (2022), Mapping Genomic Loci Implicates Genes and Synaptic Biology in Schizophrenia, *Nature*, p. 1. https://doi.org/10.1038/s41586-022-04434-5. Advance online publication. https://doi.org/10.1038/s41586-022-04434-5
104 Schizophrenia Working Group of the Psychiatric Genomics Consortium, 2022, p. 2.
105 Hellwege et al. (2017), Population Stratification in Genetic Association Studies, *Current Protocols in Human Genetics*, 95, 1.22.1–1.22.23. https://doi.org/10 .1002/cphg.48
106 Charney, 2021, p. 19.
107 Coop, G., & Przeworski, M. (2022), Lottery, Luck, or Legacy?, Published online Feb 2, 2022, p. 6. https://doi.org/10.1111/evo.14449

108 Richardson, K., & Jones, M. C. (2019), Why Genome-wide Associations with Cognitive Ability Measures are Probably Spurious, *New Ideas in Psychology,* *55,* 35–41, p. 37. https://doi.org/10.1016/j.newideapsych.2019.04.005

109 Read, J., Johnstone, L., & Taitimu, M. (2013), Psychosis, Poverty and Ethnicity, in J. Read & J. Dillon (Eds.), *Models of Madness: Psychological, Social and Biological Approaches to Psychosis* (2nd ed., pp. 191–209), London: Routledge.

110 Turkheimer E. (2016), Weak Genetic Explanation 20 Years Later: Reply to Plomin et al. (2016), *Perspectives on Psychological Science,* *11,* 24–28, p. 27. https://doi.org/10.1177/1745691615617442

111 Turkheimer, E., 2019, P-hacking in GWAS, *Blogspot, GHA Project.* www.geneticshumanagency.org/gha/p-hacking-in-gwas/

112 Andrade, C. (2021), HARKing, Cherry-picking, P-hacking, Fishing Expeditions, and Data Dredging and Mining as Questionable Research Practices, *Journal of Clinical Psychiatry,* *82*(1), 20f13804. https://doi.org/10.4088/JCP.20f13804

113 Harden, K. P. (2021), *The Genetic Lottery: Why DNA Matters for Social Equality,* Princeton, NJ: Princeton University Press, p. 62.

114 Sullivan et al. (2012), Don't Give Up On GWAS, *Molecular Psychiatry,* *17,* 2–3, p. 2. https://doi.org/10.1038/mp.2011.94

115 Turkheimer, 2019, P-hacking in GWAS.

116 Sullivan, et al. & the Psychiatric Genomics Consortium (2018), Psychiatric Genomics: An Update and an Agenda, *American Journal of Psychiatry,* *175,* 15–27. https://doi.org/10.1176/appi.ajp.2017.17030283

117 Whitaker, R. (2010), *Anatomy of an Epidemic: Magic Bullets, Psychiatric Drugs, and the Astonishing Rise of Mental Illness in America.* New York: Crown.

118 Angell M. (2000), Is Academic Medicine for Sale?, *The New England Journal of Medicine,* *342,* 1516–1518, p. 1516. https://doi.org/10.1056/NEJM200005183422009

119 Kim, et al. (2021), A Genome-wide Association Study for Concussion Risk, *Medicine and Science in Sports and Exercise,* *53,* 704–711. https://doi.org/10.1249/MSS.0000000000002529

120 Dalvie et al. (2020), Genomic Influences on Self-Reported Childhood Maltreatment, *Translational Psychiatry,* *10*(1), 38. https://doi.org/10.1038/s41398-020-0706-0

121 23andMe (2014), Genes Involved in Brain Development Influence Crying Habits: A Genome Wide Association Study. https://blog.23andme.com/wp-content/uploads/2014/10/ASHG2014_Chao_CryEasily-1.pdf

122 Burri et al. (2012), A Genome-wide Association Study of Female Sexual Dysfunction, *PLoS One,* *7*(4), e35041. https://doi.org/10.1371/journal.pone.0035041

123 May-Wilson et al. (2022), Large-scale GWAS of Food Liking Reveals Genetic Determinants and Genetic Correlations with Distinct Neurophysiological Traits, *Nature Communication,* *13,* 2743, 1–13. https://doi.org/10.1038/s41467-022-30187-w

124 Hill et al. (2019), Genome-Wide Analysis Identifies Molecular Systems and 149 Genetic Loci Associated with Income, *Nature Communications,* *10*(1), 5741. https://doi.org/10.1038/s41467-019-13585-5

125 23andMe (December 19, 2018), I Scream, You Scream, Our Genes Scream for Ice Cream! https://blog.23andme.com/23andme-research/genes-scream-for-ice-cream/

126 Song et al. (2022), Genetics, Leadership Position, and Well-Being: An Investigation with a Large-Scale GWAS, *Proceedings of the National Academy of Sciences,* *119*(12), e2114271119. https://doi.org/10.1073/pnas.2114271119

127 Day, F. R., Ong, K. K., & Perry, J. (2018), Elucidating the Genetic Basis of Social Interaction and Isolation, *Nature Communications, 9*(1), 2457. https://doi.org/10.1038/s41467-018-04930-1

128 Hu et al. (2016), GWAS of 89,283 Individuals Identifies Genetic Variants Associated with Self-Reporting of Being a Morning Person, *Nature Communications, 7*, 10448. https://doi.org/10.1038/ncomms10448

129 Niarchou et al. (2021), Genome-Wide Association Study of Musical Beat Synchronization Demonstrates High Polygenicity, BioRxiv. https://doi.org/10.1101/836197

130 Linnér et al. (2019), Genome-wide Association Analyses of Risk Tolerance and Risky Behaviors in Over One Million Individuals Identify Hundreds of Loci and Shared Genetic Influences, *Nature Genetics, 51*(2), 245–257. https://doi.org/10.1038/s41588-018-0309-3

131 van de Vegte et al. (2020), Genome-Wide Association Studies and Mendelian Randomization Analyses for Leisure Sedentary Behaviours, *Nature Communications, 11*(1), 1770. https://doi.org/10.1038/s41467-020-15553-w

132 Ganna et al. (2019), Large-Scale GWAS Reveals Insights into the Genetic Architecture of Same-Sex Sexual Behavior, *Science, 365*(6456), eaat7693. https://doi.org/10.1126/science.aat7693

133 van de Vegte et al., 2020.

134 Pirastu et al. (2015), Genome-wide Association Analysis on Five Isolated Populations Identifies Variants of the HLA-DOA Gene Associated with White Wine Liking, *European Journal of Human Genetics, 23*(12), 1717–1722. https://doi.org/10.1038/ejhg.2015.34

135 Plomin, 2018, p. vii.

136 Janssens, A. C. J. W. (2019), Validity of Polygenic Risk Scores: Are We Measuring What We Think We Are?, *Human Molecular Genetics, 28*(R2), R143–R150, p. R143. https://doi.org/10.1093/hmg/ddz205. PMID: 31504522; PMCID: PMC7013150.

137 Flint, Greenspan, & Kendler, 2020, pp. 87–88.

138 Privé et al. (2022), Portability of 245 Polygenic Scores When Derived from the UK Biobank and Applied to 9 Ancestry Groups from the Same Cohort, *American Journal of Human Genetics, 109*, 12–23. https://doi.org/10.1016/j.ajhg.2021.11.008

139 Comfort, N. (2018, September 25th), Genetic Determinism Rides Again, *Nature, 561.* https://www.nature.com/articles/d41586-018-06784-5

140 Turkheimer, E. (2019), The Social Science Blues, *Hastings Center Report, 49*(3), 45–47, p. 46. https://doi.org/10.1002/hast.1008

141 Kolker, 2020, *Hidden Valley Road: Inside the Mind of an American Family,* New York: Anchor, p. 254.

142 Burt, C. (2022), Challenging the Utility of Polygenic Scores for Social Science: Environmental Confounding, Downward Causation, and Unknown Biology (prepublication draft), *Behavioral and Brain Sciences,* 1–36, p. 23. https://doi.org/10.1017/S0140525X22001145

143 Baverstock K. (2019), Polygenic Scores: Are They a Public Health Hazard?, *Progress in Biophysics and Molecular Biology, 149*, 4–8, p. 8. https://doi.org/10.1016/j.pbiomolbio.2019.08.004

144 Plomin, 2018, p. 68.

145 Plomin, 2018, p. 165.

146 Plomin, 2018, p. 5.

147 Plomin, 2018, pp. 149–150.

148 Plomin, 2018, p. 151.

149 Plomin, 2018, p. 187.

150 Panofsky, A. (2014), *Misbehaving Science: Controversy and the Development of Behavior Genetics*, Chicago: University of Chicago Press, p. 177.
151 Okbay et al. (2022), Polygenic Prediction of Educational Attainment Within and Between Families from Genome-wide Association Analyses in 3 Million Individuals, *Nature Genetics, 54,* 437–449. https://doi.org/10.1038/s41588 -022-01016-z
152 Schork et al. (2022), Indirect Paths from Genetics to Education, *Nature Genetics, 54*(4), 372–373. https://doi.org/10.1038/s41588-021-00999-5
153 Charney, E. (2013, September 19th), Still Chasing Ghosts: A New Genetic Methodology Will Not Find the "Missing Heritability," *Independent Science News.* https://www.independentsciencenews.org/health/still-chasing-ghosts-a -new-genetic-methodology-will-not-find-the-missing-heritability/
154 Joseph, 2015, p. 220.
155 https://www.ferris.edu/HTMLS/news/jimcrow/question/2005/november.htm; https://www.pbs.org/wgbh/aia/part4/4h3106t.html
156 Feldman & Riskin, 2022.

3 Schizophrenia Family Studies

In the previous chapter, we saw that there is good reason to be skeptical of recent claims that "genes for schizophrenia" have been found, especially in the context of decades of such claims that fell by the wayside. In the next four chapters I will closely examine the evidence that researchers believe justified schizophrenia gene searches in the first place: family, twin, and adoption studies. Although the results of these studies led psychiatry long ago to declare that the "genetics of schizophrenia" debate was closed in favor of genetics, I will show in the chapters to come that there is every reason to reopen the debate.

Family Pedigrees and Family Studies

Schizophrenia genetic researcher David Rosenthal once observed, "To demonstrate that genes have anything to do with schizophrenia. ...the frequency of schizophrenia in the relatives of schizophrenics should be positively correlated with the degree of blood relationship to the schizophrenic index cases."[1] The first attempt to establish this correlation was the *family pedigree method*, which maps a family through several generations, and identifies family members affected by the trait or condition in question. The early 20th century saw many publications containing pedigree charts and descriptions of families affected by "insanity," "feeblemindedness," "genius," "criminality," pellagra, and so on.[2]

Figure 3.1 shows a five-generation 1911 family pedigree chart of the mating of a "feeble-minded" woman and an "alcoholic" man.[3] The author, Charles Davenport, was a leading eugenicist in the early part of the 20th century. Davenport and other eugenicists used such charts to support their argument that psychological traits, socially disapproved behaviors, and diseases such as pellagra show "a strong hereditary bias."[4] More recent schizophrenia pedigrees spanning several generations are seen in Jon Karlsson's 1966 book *The Biologic Basis of Schizophrenia*.[5]

Moving on from family pedigree studies, the next method of studying relatives was the *family study method*. In schizophrenia research, this method identifies a group of people diagnosed/labeled with schizophrenia, and then

DOI: 10.4324/9781003293279-3

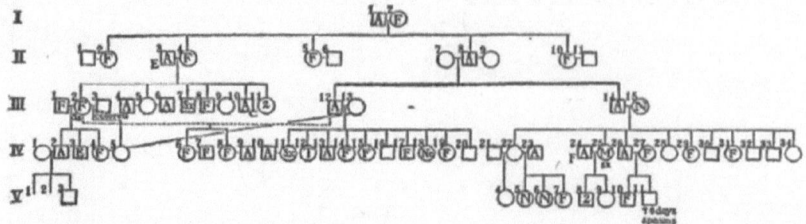

Fig. 49.—Pedigree of a Massachusetts family comprising much feeble-mindedness or imbecility, F; associated with alcoholism, A; criminality, C; sex immorality, Sx; epilepsy, E; M, migrainous; Ne, neurotic; T, tubercular. Note the association of alcoholism with imbecility.

I, 1, a basket-maker, alcoholic, married a feeble-minded woman. Of their 5 children (II, 2–10) 4 were feeble-minded and the other, II, 8, shiftless and an alcoholic. II, 4, married an epileptic alcoholic and they had 7 children. The oldest Amanda, III, 2, feeble-minded and sexually immoral, married, first, a feeble-minded man, III, 1, by whom she had 3 children, 1 alcoholic and immoral, 1 epileptic and a cripple, 1 feeble-minded; secondly, by a colored man, III, 3, she had 1 illegitimate colored child, IV, 5; thirdly, by an alcoholic, she had 2 other feeble-minded illegitimate offspring, both of whom married, the first a feeble-minded man, the second an alcoholic consumptive. The second daughter, III, 5, married twice, both alcoholics, but had no offspring; III, 7, was sexually immoral as was also the imbecile son, III, 8. III, 10, was alcoholic and criminal and two daughters, III, 11, were normal. II, 8, a shiftless alcoholic known as "Woodchuck Pete" married twice. By his first wife, a normal woman, he had two sons, both alcoholic. The oldest, III, 12, we have met above as the illegitimate husband of III, 2. He married later her daughter, IV, 4, they had 11 children. The oldest daughter, sexually immoral, IV, 11, married an alcoholic but had no children. IV, 12, was a consumptive; IV, 13, an alcoholic, and of the others, 4 are imbeciles and 1 neurotic, 4 being state wards. III, 14 married a normal woman and they had 10 children. IV, 22, married first a normal but shiftless man whom she left for non-support; her second husband was an alcoholic wanderer, by whom she had 2 normal and 1 feeble-minded child. IV, 25, migraine and immoral, married an alcoholic imbecile by whom she had 3 normal but scrofulous children. IV, 26, an alcoholic, married a feeble-minded woman and had 2 children, 1 feeble-minded, 1 died at 6 days of spasms. Of remaining 7 children, 2 are feeble-minded. F. W., 1.

Figure 3.1 1911 Family Pedigree Chart of the Mating of a "Feeble-minded" Woman and an "Alcoholic" Man

determines whether their biological relatives are diagnosed/labeled at a significantly higher level versus the biological relatives of a control group, or versus the general population expectation. If schizophrenia is found to cluster or "run" in families, the condition is familial.

"Runs in the Family" ≠ Genetic

The key point, however, is that *"familial"* does not equal *"it's genetic."* American basketball player Canyon Barry shoots free throws underhand like his father, NBA Hall of Famer Rick Barry. "Despite his father's success," a journalist wrote, the "technique dismissively known as 'Granny style' had all but disappeared. Canyon Barry knew all this when he made the switch. He knew the mockery he could expect … . Barry took the ribbing in stride."[6] Does Canyon Barry shoot free throws underhand because he is genetically predisposed to do so, or because he learned this rarely used technique from his famous father? Most people intuitively would agree that Canyon's free-throw shooting style is the result of learned behavior and his relationship with his father, but family pedigree charts and family studies can't provide an answer to this question.

In the same way, psychiatric disorders, medical conditions, and behavioral characteristics can run in families due solely to environmental factors such as exposure to common rearing patterns and abuse, trauma, learned behavior, diet, common exposure to pathogens, and many other aspects of the physical, social, and family environment. In the 2020 second edition of *How Genes Influence Behavior*, Flint, Greenspan, and Kendler recognized that a condition running in the family can be caused by the common environments families share:

> In human families, relatives can be similar because they share environments or because they share genes, or both. Relatives share all kinds of environments. They live in the same neighborhoods, often attend religious services together, eat a similar diet, are exposed to the same level of harmony or conflict in their home, and might all live close to an industrial plant that pumps out pollution into the air or water. All of these reasons and more could explain the resemblance among members of the same family.[7]

On this single point, that family study findings cannot be interpreted genetically, psychiatric geneticists and the field's critics are in agreement. And yet, as one of countless examples of mainstream media misinformation on issues related to genetics and behavior, the author of a 2016 CNN report on schizophrenia and genetics wrote, "Importantly, schizophrenia often runs in families, so scientists have long believed it is a genetic disorder."[8] A running theme of this book, and of many of my previous publications, is that the mainstream media and authoritative academic texts systematically mislead people about the methods and results of genetic research in areas of human behavior.

Ernst Rüdin and the "Munich School" of Psychiatric Genetics

Although most modern psychiatric genetic researchers understand that familial clustering of a psychiatric condition does not prove anything about genetic causes, this hasn't always been the case. To better understand this point, we must look at the roots of this field.

The First Schizophrenia Family Study

The first systematic schizophrenia family study was published in 1916 by Ernst Rüdin, the Swiss-German "father" of the psychiatric genetics field and co-founder of the German "racial hygiene" movement, and dozens more have been published since.[9] Most early studies were carried out by strong supporters of genetic causation theories, who did not diagnose/label blindly or use a control group, and who frequently diagnosed or labeled people on the basis of vague and differing definitions of schizophrenia, sometimes based on hearsay or sketchy information about unavailable or deceased relatives.

A major product of Rüdin's founding "Munich School" of psychiatric genetics was the "empirical genetic prognosis" (*empirische Erbprognose*), which involved calculating the age-corrected probability that (presumably hereditary) psychiatric conditions would eventually appear in the biological relatives and descendants of people diagnosed with these conditions. These calculations, which were based mainly on family studies, produced "morbid risk" (MR) percentage figures for various groups of relatives biologically related to the diagnosed "proband." The term *proband* is used in psychiatric genetics to represent a study's first-identified relative.

In his 1916 investigation, Rüdin studied 2,732 siblings of 755 schizophrenia (dementia praecox) patients, and calculated a narrowly defined MR of 5.4 percent, and a broadly defined MR of 7.7 percent.[10] Rüdin's colleagues and others subsequently confirmed that the age-corrected schizophrenia risks among the relatives of schizophrenia patients were higher than the rate expected in the general population, but mistakenly assumed that these elevated rates were caused by hereditary factors.

Rüdin's Suppressed Family Study of "Manic-Depressive Insanity"

Gundula Kösters and colleagues published a 2015 article on Rüdin's 1920s-era family study of "manic-depressive insanity" (now called bipolar disorder)—a study Rüdin never published.[11] They described Rüdin's unpublished manic-depression family study as consisting of "approximately 160 pages of unbound typescript, each chapter paginated separately, with Rüdin's hand-written corrections, and numerous large-format, hand-written charts."[12]

Rüdin's large manic-depression sample consisted of 661 German probands from 650 families, and included 4,351 siblings in total. In 566 families both parents were "healthy," and in 84 families one parent had an affective disorder. According to Kösters and colleagues, Rüdin compared the morbid risks he calculated in these families against "the proportions expected from a Mendelian crossing in order to prove Mendelian inheritance and thereby the inheritance of affective disorders."[13] They concluded that Rüdin decided against publishing this study because the results did not fit his theory of single-gene Mendelian inheritance, or his advocacy of eugenic policies.[14]

Rüdin and German National Socialism

In the first part of the National Socialist era (1933–1945), Rüdin played a major role in creating and implementing the German "Law for the Prevention of Genetically Diseased Offspring" (*Gesetz zur Verhütung erbkranken Nachwuchses*). Rüdin was one of three co-authors of a 1934 commentary summarizing the law's alleged scientific justification.[15] This law provided for the forced eugenic surgical sterilization of people diagnosed/labeled with schizophrenia, "manic-depressive insanity," "feeble-mindedness," and several non-psychiatric conditions. Approximately 400,000

Germans were forcibly sterilized under the law between 1934 and 1939, many based on being labeled "feeble-minded" or "schizophrenic." About 6,000 people died as a direct result of the surgical procedure.[16] Rüdin viewed the infamous 1935 anti-Semitic German Nuremburg Laws as an important scientific achievement.[17] Nevertheless, he was considered a leading figure in international scientific circles throughout the 1930s.[18]

German psychiatric geneticists of the 1930s and 1940s strongly supported compulsory sterilization and other racial hygienic (*Rassenhygiene*) measures in part because they believed that societal and racial "degeneration" would eventually result if such measures were not implemented.[19] In collaboration with his psychiatric genetic Munich right-hand men Hans Luxenburger and Bruno Schulz, much of Rüdin's National Socialist era work involved calculating psychiatric disorder morbidity risks in the service of the regime's sterilization law and other racial hygienic measures.[20] In this era Rüdin, for him at long last, found strong governmental support for the program he had developed at the beginning of his career in 1903, when he called for supporting the "maximum propagation of those who are healthy, robust and ... ethically superior," while preventing the reproduction of "the weak, ill, unfit, and morally reprehensible from reproduction by artificial selection ... by instruction and by private and government force."[21]

Luxenburger, also a strong supporter of eugenic policies and practices both before and after 1933, published his schizophrenia twin study in 1928, which was the first psychiatric twin study ever published.[22] In a 1999 article, psychiatric geneticists Alastair Cardno and Peter McGuffin wrote, "Luxenburger and Schulz opposed [eugenic] policies on both moral and scientific grounds."[23] Not true. Both Luxenburger and Schulz promoted eugenic policies in the Third Reich.[24]

From Sterilization to Killing

Hitler's regime moved beyond forced eugenic sterilization in the late 1930s and instituted a secret plan to kill mental patients and others in a program named "T4," a form of murder euphemistically referred to by the authorities as "euthanasia." The German "euthanasia" program led to the killing of approximately 70,000 people by gas, lethal injection, starvation, and other methods in the first phase between 1939 and 1941, under the direction of the government and doctors and psychiatrists.[25] Thousands more were killed between 1939 and 1945 in further "wild euthanasia" actions both in Germany and in the occupied territories. Although I am unaware of evidence that Rüdin played a role in initiating the "euthanasia" program, the evidence is clear that he helped implement and justify it, and that he participated in aspects of it.[26] It is also likely that the records from Rüdin's earlier schizophrenia family study were used to identify people to be sterilized or killed.[27]

The brains of some "euthanasia" victims were sent to Rüdin's Munich institute for evaluation and research.[28] According to his biographer Matthias Weber, "Rüdin considered the broadening of the criteria for killing handicapped newborns to be a scientific issue of importance to the war effort."[29] In 1944, Rüdin contemplated publishing an article in the journal he edited legitimizing euthanasia based on "thoroughly investigated children."[30] Clearly, at this point Rüdin still believed that Germany would win the war, and that open support in scientific journals for killing "hereditarily tainted" and "unfit" children and mental patients would become acceptable after the anticipated German victory. Rüdin chillingly wrote in 1942 that a German victory "will only inspire us…to multiply our racial hygienic efforts."[31] Fortunately for humanity, the father of psychiatric genetics never got the chance.

In a 2005 article, German psychiatric geneticist Peter Propping (1942–2016), winner of an International Society of Psychiatric Genetics "Lifetime Achievement Award," described his field's "sinister history":

> When the National Socialists came to power in Germany in 1933, the protagonists of the Munich school helped guide psychiatric genetics along the slippery slope from the sterilization of psychiatric patients to their deaths in an organized euthanasia program. Ernst Rüdin was a prominent protagonist of the German racial hygiene movement, his research program as well as his political activities being guided by the idea of a "healthy race.". … Irrespective of whether we can understand or not, however, we should never forget that eugenic theory developed through the reasoning of psychiatric genetics. [32]

For Rüdin and others, a finding that schizophrenia runs in the family ultimately led to the conclusion that "schizophrenics" must be killed.

Psychiatric Genetic Accounts of Rüdin

Details of these atrocities have been known in the English-speaking world since the 1980s and earlier.[33] There are three main categories of contemporary psychiatric genetic accounts of Rüdin and his work.[34] (1) Those who write about German psychiatric genetics in the Nazi period, but either fail to mention Rüdin at all, or cast him in a favorable light. These accounts see German psychiatric genetics as being, at most, guilty "by association."[35] (2) Those who acknowledge that Rüdin helped promote eugenic sterilization and/or may have worked with the Nazis (Rüdin became a Party member in 1937),[36] but otherwise paint a positive picture of Rüdin's research and fail to mention his participation in the "euthanasia" killing program. (3) Those who have written that Rüdin committed and supported unspeakable atrocities. Overall, as Arribas-Ayllon and colleagues concluded, "the image of Rüdin as an advocate of 'racial hygiene,' or the Munich Institute as a 'think tank' for Nazi health policy, is not part of the official birth story of psychiatric genetics."[37]

Kallmann's Study

Another early schizophrenia family study was the large 1938 investigation of 1,087 German schizophrenia patients and their 13,851 relatives. It was performed by Rüdin's psychiatric genetic colleague Franz Kallmann, who believed that his results provided "conclusive proof of the inheritance of schizophrenia."[38] This study was published in English after Kallmann had to immigrate to the United States in 1936 due to his partial Jewish ancestry—a country where many states already had passed laws permitting the compulsory eugenic sterilization of people labeled "insane" or "schizophrenic."[39] Nevertheless, as Kenneth Kendler and Astrid Klee acknowledged in a 2022 article, Kallmann continued to maintain "enthusiasm for the eugenic ideals championed by Rüdin."[40]

Kallmann reported a schizophrenia morbidity risk of 16.4 percent in the biological children of his probands, and lower rates among other types of relatives.[41] He compared these rates to the much lower general population expectation. Genetic researchers' beliefs, conclusions, and recommendations usually appear in a concluding section or chapter after they present and interpret their data, but Kallmann began the book describing his study with a chapter titled, "Genetic and Eugenic Problems in the Field of Schizophrenia." Prior to presenting his data, Kallmann called for directing eugenic measures not only at people diagnosed/labeled with schizophrenia, but at their non-diagnosed "heterozygotic taint-carrier" biological relatives as well.[42] For Kallmann, these relatives were "eugenically undesirable" people whose numbers should be "kept at the lowest possible number" by sterilization and other means.[43] While still active in Nazi Germany, Kallmann in 1935 called for the "prevention of reproduction" (forced sterilization) of "relatives of schizophrenics who stand out because of minor anomalies, and, above all, to define each of them as being undesirable from the eugenic point of view at the beginning of their reproductive years."[44]

Like Rüdin, Kallmann believed strongly that the reproduction of "schizophrenics" posed a eugenic danger to society. As the founding father of American psychiatric genetics, Kallmann, in addition to Eliot Slater, played a major role in bringing Rüdin, Luxenburger, and Schulz's Munich School message to the English-speaking world.[45] An admiring American colleague wrote of his work, "Out of Rüdin's laboratory came Kallmann and many of the other workers who developed psychiatric genetics and introduced it internationally."[46]

Upon arriving in the United States, Kallmann wrote the following in a 1938 edition of *Eugenical News*:

> From a eugenic point of view, it is particularly disastrous that these [schizophrenia] patients not only continue to crowd mental hospitals all

over the world, but also afford, to society as a whole, an unceasing source of maladjusted cranks, asocial eccentrics and the lowest types of criminal offenders. Even the faithful believer in the predominance of individual liberty will admit that mankind would be much happier without those numerous adventurers, fanatics, and pseudo-saviors of the world who are found again and again to come from the schizophrenic genotype.[47]

Because Kallmann viewed his "schizophrenic probands" and their relatives as the dangerous carriers of the "hereditary taint of schizophrenia," and because he did not diagnose/label people blindly, his objectivity has been called into question by several authors.[48] Kallmann failed to adequately describe how he defined "schizophrenia" in his 1938 family study, and as Boyle has argued, some people labeled with schizophrenia in the early European studies may actually have suffered from the viral infection *encephalitis lethargica*.[49] Others may have been, using Kallmann's own words, non-psychotic "maladjusted cranks," "asocial eccentrics," "criminal offenders," "adventurers," "fanatics," and "pseudo-saviors." Eight years later, Kallmann published a large and controversial schizophrenia twin study.[50]

Kallmann wrote a 1947 letter in support of Rüdin for the latter's denazification hearing after World War II, preposterously claiming that Rüdin "is no criminal, of course," and that "scientific and cultural progress needs men like Dr. Rüdin."[51] This description contrasted sharply with the Swiss government's judgment of Rüdin only five days after the German government's capitulation in May 1945. According to the Swiss authorities, they decided to revoke Rüdin's citizenship because his deeds "brought immense suffering and ruin for millions of innocent people":

> Rüdin belongs definitely to the intellectual leadership circle of the National Socialist regime. He was the expert who prepared the German racial-political legislation which brought immense suffering and ruin for millions of innocent people. Besides his scientific activity he...played a pronounced political role. Rüdins life's work contradicts the laws of humanity...[52]

Kallmann published a "Heredity and Eugenics" annual review in the *American Journal of Psychiatry* from 1944 until his death in 1965. Themes in these reviews included positive references to eugenic theories and policies, and the alleged benefits of the compulsory eugenic sterilization laws then existing in many U.S. states.[53]

Modern Family Studies

By the 1970s or so, most psychiatric geneticists were willing to concede the point that genetic and environmental influences cannot be disentangled in a family study, and that the proper interpretation of finding elevated schizophrenia rates among genetically related family members is that the condition is familial, but not necessarily genetic.

An example of a modern schizophrenia family study is a 1985 investigation by Kendler, Alan Gruenberg, and Ming Tsuang, who assessed the risk for psychiatric disorders among the 723 first-degree relatives of people diagnosed with schizophrenia at an Iowa psychiatric hospital, versus the risk among the 1,056 first-degree relatives of non-diagnosed matched surgical control patients. The researchers diagnosed probands and relatives blindly, using DSM-III criteria. They obtained information on relatives from personal interviews and/or hospital records. Kendler and colleagues calculated a schizophrenia "morbid risk" percentage that was significantly greater in the relatives of people diagnosed with schizophrenia (3.7%), versus the relatives of controls (0.2%). They concluded that this difference "provides strong evidence that schizophrenia, as defined by DSM-III, is a familial disorder."[54]

Like the Kendler study, several schizophrenia family studies published after 1980 used control groups and made diagnoses blindly based on structured interviews. Most found lower first-degree relative rates than the studies published prior to 1980, and at least three studies found no significant difference between the first-degree biological relatives of people diagnosed with schizophrenia versus the expected population rate, or versus the rate among the first-degree relatives of controls.[55] In the more methodologically sound modern schizophrenia family studies, the first-degree biological relatives of people diagnosed with schizophrenia were diagnosed, on average, roughly four times more often than the 1 percent rate in the general population.[56]

Irving Gottesman's Schizophrenia Risk "Figure 10"

Irving Gottesman published his subsequently widely reproduced "Figure 10" in his 1991 book *Schizophrenia Genesis*.[57] Gottesman's figure was based on schizophrenia family and twin data, and showed that the more closely someone is genetically related to a person diagnosed with schizophrenia, the greater risk that person has of being similarly diagnosed. Gottesman's figure displayed the "Grand average risk for developing schizophrenia compiled from the family and twin studies conducted in European populations between 1920 and 1987."

The risk factors Gottesman reported in his figure were as follows: "General population" = 1 percent, "Spouses of patients" = 2 percent, "First cousins (third degree)" = 2 percent, "Uncles/Aunts" = 2 percent, "Nephews/ Nieces" = 4 percent, "Grandchildren" = 5 percent, "Half siblings" = 6 percent, "Children" = 13 percent, "Siblings" = 9 percent, "Siblings with 1 schizophrenic parent " = 17 percent, "DZ twins" = 17 percent, "Parents" = 6 percent, "MZ twins" = 48 percent, "Offspring of dual matings" = 46 percent.[58] I analyzed Gottesman's schizophrenia risk factors in Chapter 6 of *The Missing Gene,* and in an article I co-authored with Jonathan Leo.[59] Here I will briefly summarize the main points from these publications.

Gottesman wrote that his figure demonstrated that the risk for schizophrenia increases proportionately as the relatives' genetic similarity increases, or as he put it, "the degree of risk correlates highly with the degree of genetic relatedness."[60] However, the risk percentages he reported also show that risks correlate roughly with the degree of *environmental* similarity shared by relatives. Gottesman's schizophrenia risk percentages cannot be interpreted genetically for these additional reasons. (1) Gottesman included methodologically unsound research based on questionable or false twin study assumptions (see Chapter 4). (2) Gottesman did not include more recent findings, and did not include studies performed outside of Europe. This meant that the risks were disproportionately weighted by the large-sample 1938 Kallmann study. (3) The twin-based risk percentages were inflated by Gottesman's use of the "proband" concordance method (see Chapter 5). (4) The twin-based risk percentages did not include much lower opposite-sex DZ concordance rates (see Chapter 5). (5) "Offspring of dual matings" studies (where both biological parents are diagnosed/labeled with schizophrenia) are problematic, and the results can be explained on non-genetic grounds.[61] (6) From the genetic perspective the DZ twin and sibling risks should be similar, but the DZ twin risk is almost twice as great as the sibling risk (17% versus 9%).

Although rarely mentioned by textbook and review article authors reproducing and discussing Gottesman's figure, the risks are consistent with a genetic *or* a purely environmental understanding of schizophrenia and psychosis. The same can be said about the family I will examine in the next section.

Hidden Valley Road

The boilerplate theme of books and articles appearing since the 1980s, popularizing behavioral genetic and psychiatric genetic research, starts with the supposedly misguided environmentalist and psychoanalytic ideas that mental disorders are sometimes caused by "refrigerator mothers" or "schizophrenogenic mothers." After bashing these strawmen, the story continues that what genetic determinists sometimes call "blank slatist" environmental theories of causation were eventually discredited by genetic researchers performing twin and adoption studies, some of whom went on to discover predisposing genes at the molecular genetic level.[62] The general theme is that objective modern science has proven environmentally focused writers and scholars wrong, and has shown that biological and genetic factors are predominant.

The Galvin Family and Schizophrenia

Continuing along these lines, in 2020 journalist Robert Kolker published *Hidden Valley Road: Inside the Mind of an American Family* (abbreviated as HVR).[63] This was the story of a real mid-20th century "baby boom"

Caucasian-American middle-class family of 14. Don and Mimi Galvin had 12 children, born between 1945 and 1965. Remarkably, the first ten children in this Colorado family were male, and the final two were female. This is how Stephen Rodrick of *Rolling Stone* described the Galvin family:

> On the surface, the Galvins were a postwar American dream. Don was a World War II veteran helping to jump-start the just-opened Air Force Academy in Colorado Springs alongside his witty and selfless wife. The first 10 Galvin kids, born beginning in 1945, were handsome boys who became high school football and hockey stars in their growing boomtown. Two beautiful daughters, Lindsay and Margaret, followed them. The Galvins lived on the outskirts of the city, on Hidden Valley Road, and were the envy of other families throughout Colorado Springs.[64]

Of the ten boys, six were eventually diagnosed with schizophrenia. They also were diagnosed with other psychiatric disorders. Kolker recognized that "these brothers were all different and manifested their illnesses differently."[65] Although psychiatry lumped the brothers' differing behavioral patterns under the "schizophrenia" umbrella, we could easily conclude that they experienced six *different* "illnesses."

A major reason why Kolker believed that the case for genetic explanations was airtight, and that family dynamics explanations were weak or discredited, was that the Danish-American adoption studies of the 1960s (and after) had confirmed the earlier "gold standard" findings from twin research.[66] Kolker believed that these adoption studies showed that family environments play little if any role in causing schizophrenia or psychosis. I will closely examine the supposed "gold standard" twin studies in Chapters 4 and 5, and the problematic Danish-American adoption studies in Chapter 6.

The HVR story is remarkable, tragic, and anger provoking, yet we have seen that "running in the family" does not equal "genetic," because families share a common environment as well as common genes. Kolker described how sexual abuse was rampant in this family, both from inside the family and outside the family. There was no escaping it. For the youngest child Lindsay, "it seemed as if" the second-born Galvin child Jim "had taken [sexual] liberties with every young child around him."[67] In addition, Mimi believed that a trusted Catholic priest had been sexually "pursuing her boys like boxes of cereal at the supermarket until he found the one he liked the best. 'He had culled my family,' she said. 'He knew it was a big family of boys.'"[68]

So now we have identified sexual abuse as a massive, powerful nongenetic source of psychological distress and "psychopathology" in the Galvin family. And yet for Kolker it's *genes* that tell the story of this family, stating flatly, "Sexual abuse does not cause schizophrenia. That much is certain. Even a torrent of sexual abuse like what Mimi had envisioned still could not answer the bigger question of why there had been so much mental ill-ness in their family."[69] A *torrent* of sexual abuse. Kolker went further and declared, "to be sure, no studies have ever suggested that abuse does cause schizophrenia."[70] Who was telling him such things?

The Galvin sons also were abused by the psychiatric establishment. At one point Peter Galvin was taking *six* different prescribed neuroleptic (anti-psychotic) drugs at the same time: Geodon, Risperidone, Risperdal Consta (an injectable drug), Zyprexa, Prolixin, and Thorazine.[71] Jim and Joe Galvin, at the age of fifty-three, both died from a condition known as "neuroleptic malignant syndrome," which refers to poisoning due to years of taking prescribed neuroleptic drugs.[72] According to Kolker, Mimi "had no compunction about saying that Jim and Joe both died of the medicine that was supposed to help them."[73]

Enter Robert Freedman and Lynn DeLisi

Kolker dismissed the harmful psychological impact of being a victim of trauma and sexual abuse, while downplaying the fact that reared-together siblings can influence each other's behavior, and do not develop psychosis independently of each other. He championed the work of two psychiatric researchers who supposedly had helped uncover schizophrenia's biologi-cal/genetic roots. The two were Robert Freedman, who pinned hopes on the CHRNA7 gene, and Lynn DeLisi, who focused on the SHANK2 gene. Freedman "was on the hunt for a physiological understanding of" schizo-phrenia, whereas DeLisi "wanted to track down the genetic components of schizophrenia."[74] Kolker presented these researchers' work as though they were detectives working on a cold-case murder investigation, not as researchers attempting to identify "genes for schizophrenia" that may or may not exist.

Undoubtedly, Freedman and DeLisi were motivated by a desire to prevent and better treat human suffering and dysfunction, but we saw in Chapter 2 that the winners of the "genes for schizophrenia" hunt also stand to receive professional honors, and to reap financial rewards. Freedman told Kolker that he was an "unpaid advisor" to the drug companies, but he stood to profit from patents and royalties if his nicotinic receptor drug came to mar-ket.[75] All well and good, but potential conflicts of interest and financial motivations should be completely transparent as we attempt to evaluate various schizophrenia treatment and gene discovery claims.

The CHRNA7 Gene

Kolker portrayed Freedman and DeLisi as schizophrenia gene discoverers who helped seal the case against environmental causes. We saw in Chapter 2 that the "candidate gene" era in psychiatric genetic research was a "flop," yet Kolker wrote that in 1997, "Freedman identified CHRNA7 as the first gene ever to be definitively associated with schizophrenia. He and his colleagues made history."[76] Apparently, Kolker was unaware of the 2015 psychiatric genetics candidate gene postmortem report penned by leading researchers who concluded, in relation to CHRNA7 and other schizophrenia candidate genes, "We can state with high confidence that the large common variant genetic effects originally reported in many initial candidate gene studies are highly unlikely to be true."[77]

The SHANK2 Gene

Turning to DeLisi's SHANK2 gene, the numerous publications on schizophrenia molecular genetic research rarely mention it. If SHANK2 were a true gene discovery, we would expect it to be highlighted in these publications. In a biologically oriented 2022 review article on schizophrenia, appearing in *The Lancet*, there was no mention of SHANK2 (or CHRNA7).[78] A May 2022 PubMed search for the combined terms "SHANK2" and "schizophrenia" returned only eight articles using both terms since the publication of a 2016 article DeLisi co-authored on the topic.[79] In the 2011 and (most recent) 2017 editions of her popular book *100 Questions & Answers About Schizophrenia: Painful Minds*, despite devoting many pages to genetics, DeLisi did not say anything about SHANK2.[80] Scientists usually mention their discoveries in the books they write.

DeLisi published an academic journal article on schizophrenia genetics in 2022, where she wrote of gene discovery in multiplex families like the Galvins as a goal for future research, but not as a something that had been achieved. (In "multiplex" families, multiple individuals are affected by a specific disease or condition.) Toward the end of her long career in psychiatric genetic research, DeLisi could not lay claim to any gene discoveries in multiplex families:

> Unfortunately, so many gaps exist in our understanding of normal brain development and variation, that it is difficult to put together this puzzle in its complete form so far by finding unique mutations in multiplex families.[81]

DeLisi mentioned Kolker and *Hidden Valley Road* in this 2022 article, writing that Kolker "suggests with some 'literary license' that science has made lots of progress." Perhaps DeLisi's use of the term "literary license" was a polite way of saying that Kolker's claims were overblown. DeLisi said that Kolker "describes how several years of persistent research on this family paid off with the finding that a mutation in the SHANK-2 gene appeared to be present in all the affected individuals," but she distanced herself from Kolker's description. DeLisi wrote that SHANK2 was also found in the "unaffected mother" (Mimi Galvin), and later was "found to be present in one of the unaffected female siblings and her female offspring...All three of the females had a previous lifetime history of major depression, but none had a psychosis."[82] The source DeLisi gave for these findings was "DeLisi, unpublished data," and the question then becomes why these findings were not published. The SHANK2 theory that DeLisi saw as inconclusive, Kolker presented to the world as the likely "mutation responsible for the [Galvin] family illness."[83]

DeLisi ended her 2022 article by asserting her belief that while progress has been made, there is a long way to go:

> While only one family with schizophrenia, this documentary by Robert Kolker illustrates how far we have come in attempts to define abnormalities of thinking and perception, diagnosed as schizophrenia and indicates how far we yet have to go to meet the goal of re-defining schizophrenia in the next half century.[84]

In Chapter 6 I will show that although Kolker, DeLisi, and Freedman believed that the Danish-American adoption studies played a key role in establishing schizophrenia as a genetic disorder, they did not appear to understand how these studies were performed.

Genetic Insider Accounts

Kolker did provide some interesting insights into how schizophrenia molecular genetic researchers privately viewed their results, based on conversations and interviews he had with them. DeLisi favored the approach of looking for schizophrenia genes in multiplex families like the Galvins, whereas the GWAS approach compares genes among large groups of diagnosed and non-diagnosed people. DeLisi shared her thoughts about GWAS with Kolker. "I don't believe that these hundred genes or markers are going to lead to anything," she told him.[85] Kolker earlier described GWAS investigations as a "blistering disappointment," leading the Broad Institute to "double down" and resolve "to build a bigger and better GWAS."[86] The disconnect between private "blistering disappointment" and public discovery claims and dauntless optimism is stunning, as the issue now seems more related to protecting salaries and funding, the possibility of striking it rich with drug patents and direct-to-consumer tests, reputations, being published in prestigious journals, and a refusal to recognize the possibility that one's life's work has been in vain.

Polygenic risk scores "tried to make lemonade out of lemons," the journalist Kolker wrote, and PRS researchers were merely "lumping together trivialities into something only slightly less trivial."[87] We saw in Chapter 2 that in an interview, veteran psychiatric genetic researcher Elliot Gershon described PRS to Kolker as "sort of a mindless score," and that "you can't really tell anything from the polygenic risk factor."[88]

* * *

The HVR story is worthy of book-length coverage, though from a radically different perspective than the one Kolker presented. The author told the usual story of supposedly misguided environmental theories being overturned by the twin and adoption studies I will examine in the next three chapters, subsequently crowned by scientists' discovery of the genes that cause schizophrenia. Stories of discovery sell books and possible future movie deals. Stories of disappointment and failure usually do not. Overall, despite some glimpses into the tragic world of a family riddled with abuse and dysfunction, in addition to glimpses into the behind-the-scenes world of molecular genetics insiders, Kolker's book reproduced psychiatry's long-running yet problematic "genetics of schizophrenia" story. Kolker presented a story of heroic and inspired medical science making historic gene discoveries. Others might see the "genes for schizophrenia" story as a half-century-long train wreck.

Summary and Conclusions

In this chapter I took only a brief look at schizophrenia family studies, because all sides of the "genetics of schizophrenia" debate agree that schizophrenia family study results can be explained by either nature or nurture influences. There is broad agreement, then, that family studies cannot be interpreted genetically. This is also seen in Irving Gottesman's famous 1991 schizophrenia risk percentage figure, whose results also can be explained on environmental grounds. I explored the origins of the psychiatric genetics field in Germany, and how this field was involved in many of the crimes committed by the National Socialist regime. I looked at the massive schizophrenia family study by Franz Kallmann, and described the findings of the more methodologically sound modern family studies. Finally, I reviewed a 2020 book about a family in which six children grew up to experience psychosis.

Because it is now widely understood that the results of family studies can be explained entirely by non-genetic (environmental) factors, genetic researchers and textbook authors usually cite twin studies and adoption studies as supplying key evidence in support of genetic theories of schizophrenia. While conceding the point that genetic interpretations of family study results are confounded by environmental factors, they argue for the most part that genetic interpretations of twin study and adoption study results are not. Over the next three chapters, I will challenge these positions. I begin with a critical analysis of twin research, which a leading twin researcher once referred to as the "Rosetta Stone" of behavioral genetics.[89]

Notes

1 Rosenthal, D. (1974), The Genetics of Schizophrenia, in S. Arieti & E. Brody (Eds.), *American Handbook of Psychiatry* (2nd ed., pp. 588-600), New York: Basic Books, p. 589.

2 Pedigree charts used to support eugenic claims are found, among other places, in Davenport, C. B. (2011), *Heredity in Relation to Eugenics*, New York: Henry Holt and Company.

3 Davenport, 1911, p. 84.

4 Davenport, 1911, p. 83; Davenport, C. B., & Muncey, E. B. (1916), The Hereditary Factor in Pellagra, *Eugenics Record Office Bulletin No. 16*, Cold Spring Harbor, New York. For more on early claims that pellagra was a hereditary disease, see Joseph, J. (2006), *The Missing Gene: Psychiatry, Heredity, and the Fruitless Search for Genes*, New York: Algora, Chapter 4.

5 Karlsson, J. L. (1966), *The Biologic Basis of Schizophrenia*, Springfield, IL: Charles Thomas.

6 Casey, T. (2017, February 8th), Like Father, Like Son, Like Granny? A Case for Underhand Free Throws, *New York Times*. https://www.nytimes.com/2017/02/08/sports/ncaabasketball/underhand-free-throw-rick-barry.html

7 Flint, J., Greenspan, R. J., & Kendler, K. S. (2020), *How Genes Influence Behavior* (2nd ed.), Oxford, UK: Oxford University Press, p. 11.

8 Scutti, S. (2016, October 19th), Scientists Confirm Genetics of Schizophrenia, *CNN*. https://www.cnn.com/2016/10/19/health/schizophrenia-genome-study/

9 Rüdin, E. (1916), *Zur Vererbung und Neuentstehung der Dementia Praecox* [On the Heredity and New Development of Dementia Praecox], Berlin: Springer Verlag OHG. David Rosenthal called Rüdin the "father of psychiatric genetics," see Rosenthal, D. (1981), Genetic Transmission in Schizophrenia, in S. Matthysse (Ed.), *Psychiatry and the Biology of the Human Brain: A Symposium Dedicated to Seymour S. Kety* (pp. 227–238), Elsevier, p. 227.

10 Kendler, K. S., & Zerbin-Rüdin, E. (1996), Abstract and Review of "Studien Über Vererbung und Entstehung Geistiger Storungen. I. Zur Vererbung und Neuentstehung der Dementia praecox" (Studies on the Inheritance and Origin of Mental Illness: I. To the Problem of the Inheritance and Primary Origin of Dementia Praecox), *American Journal of Medical Genetics (Neuropsychiatric Genetics), 67*, 338–342. https://doi.org/10.1002/(SICI)1096-8628(19960726)67:4<338::AID-AJMG4>3.0.CO;2-I

11 Kösters et al. (2015), Ernst Rüdin's Unpublished 1922–1925 Study "Inheritance of Manic-Depressive Insanity": Genetic Research Findings Subordinated to Eugenic Ideology, *PLoS Genetics, 11*(11), e1005524. https://doi.org/10.1371/journal.pgen.1005524

12 Kösters et al., 2015, p. 3.

13 Kösters et al., 2015, p. 5.

14 As I showed in Chapter 10 of *The Missing Gene*, the widespread claim that bipolar disorder is "highly heritable" is based on a body of weak evidence, based mainly on very problematic twin and adoption studies.

15 Gütt, A., Rüdin, E., & Ruttke, F. (1934), *Gesetz zur Verhütung Erbkranken Nachwuchses* [Law for the Prevention of Genetically Diseased Offspring], Munich: J. F. Lehmanns.

16 Schneider, F. (2011), Psychiatry Under National Socialism: Remembrance and Responsibility, *European Archives of Psychiatry and Clinical Neuroscience, 261*, Supplement 2, S111–118. https://doi.org/10.1007/s00406-011-0243-1

17 Joseph, J., & Wetzel, N. (2013), Ernst Rüdin: Hitler's Racial Hygiene Mastermind, *Journal of the History of Biology, 46*, 1–30. https://doi.org/10.1007/s10739-012-9344-6; Ploetz, A., & Rüdin, E. (1938), Zur Entwicklung des Deutschen Reichs seit der Machtübernahme unseres Führers am 30. Januar 1933 [On the Development of the German Reich since our Führer's Seizure of Power on January 30, 1933], *Archiv für Rassen- und Gesellschaftsbiologie, 32*(2), 185–186.

18 Roelcke, V. (2010), Medicine During the Nazi Period: Historical Facts and Some Implications for Teaching Medical Ethics and Professionalism, in S. Rubenfeld

(Ed.), *Medicine after the Holocaust: From the Master Race to the Human Genome and Beyond* (pp. 18–27), New York: Palgrave Macmillan.

19 Roelcke, V. (2006), Funding the Scientific Foundations of Race Policies: Ernst Rüdin and the Impact of Career Resources on Psychiatric Genetics, ca 1910–1945, in W. Eckart (Ed.), *Man, Medicine, and the State: The Human Body as an Object of Government Sponsored Medical Research in the 20th Century* (pp. 73–87), Stuttgart: Steiner; Schulze, T. G., Fangerau, H., & Propping, P. (2004), From Degeneration to Genetic Susceptibility, from Eugenics to Genetics, from Bezugsziffer to LOD Score: The History of Psychiatric Genetics, *International Review of Psychiatry*, 16, 260–283. https://doi.org/10.1080 /09540260400014419; Weindling, P. (1989), *Health, Race, and German Politics Between National Unification and Nazism, 1870-1945*, Cambridge: Cambridge University Press.

20 Joseph & Wetzel, 2013; Luxenburger, H. (1934), "Rassenhygienisch Wichtige Probleme und Ergebnisse der Zwillingspathologie" [Racial Hygienic Important Problems and Results of Twin Pathology], in E. Rüdin (Ed.), *Erblehre und Rassenhygiene im Völkischen Staat* [Genetics and Racial Hygiene in the Völkish State] (pp. 303–316), Munich: Lehmanns; Schulz, B. (1934), Rassenhygienische Eheberatung [Racial Hygienic Marriage Counseling], *Volk und Rasse, 9*, 138–143. For a detailed description of the work of Rüdin, Luxenburger, and Schulz in the Nazi era, see Weiss, S. F. (2010), *The Nazi Symbiosis: Human Genetics and Politics in the Third Reich*, Chicago: University of Chicago Press, Chapter 3.

21 Quoted in Weber, M. M. (1996), Ernst Rüdin, 1874–1952: A German Psychiatrist and Geneticist, *American Journal of Medical Genetics (Neuropsychiatric Genetics)*, 67, 323–331, p. 325. https://doi.org/10.1002/(SICI)1096-8628(19960726)67:4<323::AID-AJMG2>3.0.CO;2-N

22 Luxenburger, H. (1931), Psychiatrische Erbprognose und Eugenik [Psychiatric Genetic Prognosis and Eugenics], *Eugenik, 1*, 117–124; Luxenburger, 1934. For further documentation of Hans Luxenburger's strong support for eugenic and racial hygienic policies, both before and after 1933, see Joseph, J. (2004), *The Gene Illusion: Genetic Research in Psychiatry and Psychology under the Microscope*, New York: Algora, Chapter 2.

23 Cardno, A., & McGuffin, P. (1999), Psychiatric Genetics, in H. Freeman (Ed.), *A Century of Psychiatry* (pp. 343–347), London: Moseby, p. 344.

24 Joseph, 2004; Joseph & Wetzel, 2013; Weiss, 2010. Luxenburger, 1934; Schulz, 1934.

25 Lifton, R. J. (1986), *The Nazi Doctors*, New York: Basic Books; Proctor, R. N. (1988), *Racial Hygiene: Medicine under the Nazis*, Cambridge, MA: Harvard University Press.

26 For evidence showing Rüdin's involvement in the T4 "euthanasia" program, see Joseph & Wetzel, 2013; Müller-Hill, B. (1998), *Murderous Science*, Plainview, NY: Cold Spring Harbor Laboratory Press (original English version published in 1988); Roelcke, V. (2000), Psychiatrische Wissenschaft im Kontext Nationalsozialistischer Politik und 'Euthanasie': Zur Rolle von Ernst Rüdin und der Deutschen Forschungsanstalt/Kaiser-Wilhelm-Institut für Psychiatrie [Psychiatric Science in the Context of National Socialist Politics and "Euthanasia": On the Role of Ernst Rüdin and the German Research Institute/Kaiser-Wilhelm Institute for Psychiatry], in D. Kaufmann (Ed.), *Die Kaiser-Wilhelm-Gesellschaft im Nationalsozialismus* [The Kaiser-Wilhelm Society Under National Socialism] (pp. 112–150), Göttingen, Germany: Wallstein; Weiss, 2010.

27 Gejman, P. V. (1997), Ernst Rüdin and Nazi Euthanasia: Another Stain on His Career [Letter to the Editor], *American Journal of Human Genetics (Neuropsychiatric Genetics)*, 74, 455–456. https://doi.org/10.1002/(sici)1096-8628(19970725)74:4<455::aid-ajmg22>3.0.co;2-g; Baron, M. (1998), Psychiatric

Genetics and Prejudice: Can the Science Be Separated from the Scientist?, *Molecular Psychiatry, 3,* 96–100. https://www.nature.com/articles/4000381.pdf
28 Weiss, 2010, p. 183.
29 Weber, M. M. (2000), Psychiatric Research and Science Policy in Germany: The History of the *Deutsche Forschungsanstalt für Psychiatrie* (German Institute for Psychiatric Research) in Munich from 1917 to 1945, *History of Psychiatry, 11,* 235–258, p. 255. https://doi.org/10.1177/0957154X0001104301
30 Quoted in Weiss, 2010, p. 179.
31 Rüdin, E. (1942), Zehn Jahre Nationalsozialistischer Staat [Ten Years of the National Socialist State], *Archiv für Rassen- und Gesellschaftsbiologie, 36,* 321–322, p. 322. My translation.
32 Propping, P. (2005), The Biography of Psychiatric Genetics: From Early Achievements to Historical Burden, from an Anxious Society to Critical Geneticist, *American Journal of Medical Genetics, Part B (Neuropsychiatric Genetics), 136B (1),* 2–7, p. 3. https://doi.org/10.1002/ajmg.b.30188
33 Lifton, R. J. (1986), *The Nazi Doctors,* New York: Basic Books; Müller-Hill, 1998; Proctor, 1988.
34 Joseph & Wetzel, 2013.
35 For an example of the "guilt by association" argument, see Farmer, A., & McGuffin, P. (1999), Ethics and Psychiatric Genetics, in S. Bloch et al. (Eds.), *Psychiatric Ethics* (pp. 479–493), Oxford: Oxford University Press, p. 483.
36 Proctor, 1988.
37 Arribas-Ayllon, M., Bartlett, A., & Lewis, J. (2019), *Psychiatric Genetics: From Hereditary Madness to Big Biology,* London: Routledge, p. 53.
38 Kallmann, F. J. (1938), *The Genetics of Schizophrenia: A Study of Heredity and Reproduction in the Families of 1,087 Schizophrenics,* New York: J. J. Augustin, p. xiv.
39 Chase, A. (1980), *The Legacy of Malthus: The Social Costs of the New Scientific Racism,* Urbana, IL/Chicago: University of Illinois Press (originally published in 1977); Reilly, P. R. (1991), *The Surgical Solution: A History of Involuntary Sterilization in the United States,* Baltimore: Johns Hopkins University Press.
40 Kendler, K. S., & Klee, A. (2022), The Place of Franz Kallmann's 1938 "The Genetics of Schizophrenia" in the History of Psychiatric Genetics, *American Journal of Medical Genetics, Part B, Neuropsychiatric Genetics 189,* 26–36, p. 26. https://doi.org/10.1002/ajmg.b.32886
41 Kallmann, 1938, *The Genetics of Schizophrenia,* p. 265.
42 Kallmann, 1938, *The Genetics of Schizophrenia,* p. 3.
43 Kallmann, 1938, *The Genetics of Schizophrenia,* p. 47.
44 Quoted in Müller-Hill, 1998, p. 11.
45 Baron, 1998; Gershon, E. S. (1981), The Historical Context of Franz Kallmann and Psychiatric Genetics, *Archives of Psychiatry and Neurological Sciences, 229,* 273–276.
46 Erlenmeyer-Kimling, E. (1972), Comments on Past and Present in Genetic Research on Schizophrenia, *Psychiatric Quarterly, 46,* 363–370, p. 363.
47 Kallmann, F. J. (1938), Heredity, Reproduction, and Eugenic Procedure in the Field of Schizophrenia, *Eugenical News, 13,* 105–113, p. 105.
48 Pastore, N. (1949), The Genetics of Schizophrenia: A Special Review, *Psychological Bulletin, 46,* 285–302. https://doi.org/10.1037/h0057232
49 Boyle, M. (2002), *Schizophrenia: A Scientific Delusion?* (2nd ed.), Hove, UK: Routledge, pp. 69–76, 172–173. For an early critique of Kallmann's 1938 family study, see Pastore, 1949.
50 Kallmann, F. J. (1946), The Genetic Theory of Schizophrenia: An Analysis of 691 Schizophrenic Twin Index Families, *American Journal of Psychiatry, 103,* 309–322. https://doi.org/10.1176/ajp.103.3.309

51 Gottesman, I. I., & Bertelsen, A. (1996), Legacy of German Psychiatric Genetics: Hindsight is always 20/20, *American Journal of Medical Genetics (Neuropsychiatric Genetics)*, *67*, 317–322, p. 321. https://doi.org/10.1002/(SICI)1096-8628(19960726)67:4<317::AID-AJMG1>3.0.CO;2-J

52 Weingart, P., Kroll, J., & Bayertz, K. (1988), *Rasse, Blut und Gene: Geschichte der Eugenik und Rassenhygiene in Deutschland* [Race, Blood and Genes: History of Eugenics and Racial Hygiene in Germany], Frankfurt am Main: Suhrkamp, p. 569. Translation from Joseph & Wetzel, 2013.

53 For example, Kallmann, F. J. (1947), Review of Psychiatric Progress 1946: Heredity and Eugenics, *American Journal of Psychiatry*, *103*, 513–515; Kallmann, F. J. (1951), Review of Psychiatric Progress 1950: Heredity and Eugenics, *American Journal of Psychiatry*, *107*, 503–507.

54 Kendler, K. S., Gruenberg, A. M., & Tsuang, M. T. (1985), Psychiatric Illness in First-Degree Relatives of Schizophrenic and Surgical Control Patients, *Archives of General Psychiatry*, *42*, 770–779, p. 775. https://doi.org/10.1001/archpsyc.1985.01790310032004

55 For schizophrenia family studies finding no significant elevation of schizophrenia among first-degree biological relatives, see Abrams, R., & Taylor, M. A. (1983), The Genetics of Schizophrenia: A Reassessment Using Modern Criteria, *American Journal of Psychiatry*, *140*, 171–175. https://doi.org/10.1176/ajp.140.2.171; Coryell, W., & Zimmerman, M. (1988), The Heritability of Schizophrenia and Schizoaffective Disorders, *Archives of General Psychiatry*, *45*, 323–327. https://doi.org/10.1001/archpsyc.1988.01800280033005; Pope et al. (1982), Failure to Find Evidence of Schizophrenia in First-Degree Relatives of Schizophrenic Probands, *American Journal of Psychiatry*, *139*, 826–828. https://doi.org/10.1176/ajp.139.6.826

56 For more on modern schizophrenia family studies, see Joseph, 2006, Chapter 6; Joseph, J., & Leo, J. (2006), Genetic Relatedness and the Lifetime Risk for Being Diagnosed with Schizophrenia: Gottesman's 1991 Figure 10 Reconsidered, *Journal of Mind and Behavior*, *27*, 73–89.

57 Gottesman, I. I. (1991), *Schizophrenia Genesis*, New York: W. H. Freeman & Company, p. 96.

58 Gottesman, 1991, p. 96.

59 Joseph, 2006; Joseph & Leo, 2006.

60 Gottesman, 1991, p. 96.

61 Joseph, 2006, pp. 1215–127.

62 Pinker, S. (2002), *The Blank Slate*, New York: Viking.

63 Kolker, 2020, *Hidden Valley Road: Inside the Mind of an American Family*. New York: Anchor.

64 Rodrick, S. (2020, Aril 21st), Inside the Bestselling Medical Mystery "Hidden Valley Road," *Rolling Stone*. https://www.rollingstone.com/culture/culture-features/hidden-valley-road-robert-kolker-interview-986091/

65 Garcia-Navarro, L. (2020, April 5th), In "Hidden Valley Road," A Family's Journey Helps Shift the Science of Mental Illness, *NPR*. https://www.npr.org/2020/04/05/826695581/in-hidden-valley-road-a-familys-journey-helps-shift-the-science-of-mental-illnes

66 Kolker, 2020, Chapter 14; the "gold standard" quote is found on p. 75.

67 Kolker, 2020, p. 235.

68 Kolker, 2020, p. 241.

69 Kolker, 2020, p. 241.

70 Kolker, 2020, p. 194.

71 Kolker, 2020, p. 258.

72 Kolker, 2020, pp. 261, 264.

73 Kolker, 2020, p. 283.

74 Kolker, 2020, p. 178.
75 Kolker, 2020, pp. 246–247.
76 Kolker, 2020, p. 248.
77 Farrell et al. (2015), Evaluating Historical Candidate Genes for Schizophrenia, *Molecular Psychiatry*, 20, 555–562, pp. 556, 560. https://doi.org/10.1038/mp.2015.16
78 Jauhar, S., Johnstone, M., & McKenna, P. J. (2022), Schizophrenia, *Lancet*, 399, 473–486. https://doi.org/10.1016/S0140-6736(21)01730-X
79 Homann et al. (2016), Whole-genome Sequencing in Multiplex Families with Psychoses Reveals Mutations in the SHANK2 and SMARCA1 Genes Segregating with Illness, *Molecular Psychiatry*, 21, 1690–1695. https://doi.org/10.1038/mp.2016.24
80 DeLisi, L. E. (2011), *100 Questions & Answers About Schizophrenia: Painful Minds* (2nd ed.), Sudbury, MA: Jones & Bartlett; DeLisi, L. E. (2017), *100 Questions & Answers About Schizophrenia: Painful Minds* (3rd ed.), Burlington, MA: Jones & Bartlett.
81 DeLisi, L. E. (2022), Redefining Schizophrenia Through Genetics: A Commentary on 50 Years Searching for Biological Causes, *Schizophrenia Research*, 242, 22–24, pp. 23–24. https://doi.org/10.1016/j.schres.2021.11.017
82 DeLisi, 2022, p. 24.
83 Kolker, 2020, p. 272.
84 DeLisi, 2022, p. 24.
85 Kolker, 2020, p. 255.
86 Kolker, 2020, p. 254.
87 Kolker, 2020, p. 254.
88 Kolker, 2020, p. 254.
89 Bouchard, T. J., Jr. (1999), Foreword, in N. Segal, *Entwined Lives: Twins and What They Tell Us About Human Behavior* (pp. ix–x), New York: Dutton, p. ix.

4 A Critique of the Classical Twin Method

In this chapter, I will show that contrary to what most people have read or heard, studies of human behavior using the *classical twin method* (or "twin method") cannot be interpreted genetically. In the following chapter, I will explore the schizophrenia twin study literature in this context. Building on the writings of nearly a century of twin research critics, I will show that the main assumption these studies are based upon is false—an argument I have developed in books, peer-reviewed articles, and online articles since 1998.[1]

Twin studies supply the evidence most often cited in support of behavioral "heritability." Yet genetic interpretations of behavioral twin studies, including areas such as IQ, personality, criminality (antisocial behavioral), schizophrenia, and depression are based on the acceptance of an assumption that is clearly wrong. This is the most frequent criticism of the schizophrenia twin studies I will discuss in Chapter 5.

The twin method compares the behavioral resemblance of reared-together MZ (monozygotic, identical) versus reared-together same-sex DZ pairs (dizygotic, fraternal). MZ pairs are assumed to share a 100 percent of their segregating genes, whereas DZ pairs are assumed to share an average 50 percent of their segregating genes. This assumption has been called into question, and MZ twins might not be genetically identical, as twin researchers previously assumed.[2] Twin method results usually show that, at a statistically significant level, MZ pairs behave more alike, or correlate higher on psychological tests, compared with same-sex DZ pairs. I will designate this finding "$rMZ > rDZ$" (with r representing the behavioral correlation).

The "Equal Environment Assumption" (EEA)

As seen in Table 4.1, genetic interpretations of behavioral twin studies depend on the acceptance of several key assumptions.

We saw that Assumption #2 in Table 4.1 has been called into question, and Assumption #3 is generally true today, but less so in studies appearing prior to the 1970s. Assumptions #4 and #5 are not always fulfilled, and Assumption #6 will be discussed later. Although critics have highlighted numerous twin method problems and biases relating to sampling, diagnoses, tests used, the

DOI: 10.4324/9781003293279-4

Table 4.1 Behavioral Twin Studies and Their Assumptions

The "Classical Twin Method" Compares the Behavioral Resemblance of MZ versus Same-Sex DZ Twin Pairs

---

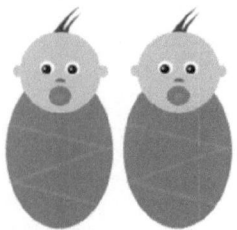

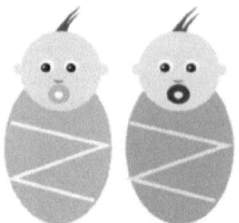

MZ Pairs
(Monozygotic, identical)
Reared together in the same family
   home

Same-Sex DZ Pairs
(Dizygotic, fraternal)
Reared together in the same family
   home

Key Assumptions

1. There exist only two types of twin pairs, monozygotic (MZ) and dizygotic (DZ).
2. MZ pairs share 100 percent of their segregating genes; DZ pairs share on average 50 percent of their segregating genes.
3. Investigators are able to reliably distinguish between MZ and DZ twin pairs (zygosity determination).
4. The psychiatric diagnosis or behavioral characteristic is found in similar numbers, or mean psychological test scores are similar (e.g., IQ, personality), among twins and non-twins (generalizability).
5. The prevalence of the psychiatric diagnosis or behavioral characteristic, or the mean psychological test score, is similar among individual MZ twins as a population, versus individual DZ twins as a population.
6. Parents of twins mate randomly for the behavioral characteristic in question (there is no "assortative mating").
7. MZ and same-sex DZ pairs grow up experiencing equal environments (the "Equal Environment Assumption," or "EEA").

If the above assumptions are true, and if the behavioral characteristic or psychiatric condition in question is valid and can be reliably identified, rMZ > rDZ is attributed to genetic factors

---

use of age-correction methods, and researcher genetic bias, here I will focus on the MZ-DZ "equal environment assumption," also known as the "EEA." The EEA has been, by far, the most controversial twin method assumption (Assumption #7 in Table 4.1), and is the key assumption in schizophrenia twin research. According to the EEA, MZ and DZ pairs grow up experiencing roughly equal environments, and the only behaviorally relevant factor distinguishing these pairs is their differing degree of *genetic* relationship to each other (100% versus an average 50%). As one group of twin researchers observed, the EEA "is crucial to everything that follows from twin research."[3]

The twin method/EEA debate remains vibrant, despite statements by criminology twin researcher J. C. Barnes and colleagues in 2014 that the debate "has been settled" in favor of the EEA's validity, and that the arguments of critics were "refuted" long ago.[4] Interestingly, in a supposedly settled debate, Barnes and colleagues responded at length to an article by fellow criminologists Callie Burt and Ronald Simons, a response that required the collaboration of no fewer than 24 people.[5]

Defining the EEA

From the twin method's inception in the 1920s until the mid-1960s, twin researchers assumed—without adding any qualifying statements—that MZ and same-sex DZ pairs grow up experiencing roughly equal environments.[6] Here I cite two examples of this "traditional" EEA definition, by twin researchers Horatio Newman and colleagues in 1937, and by schizophrenia twin researcher Einar Kringlen in 1967.

> The [twin] method ... assum[es] that environmental differences are the same for both identical and fraternal twins.[7]

> The basic underlying assumption for the classical twin method is, of course, that environmental conditions of monozygotic twins do not differ from those of dizygotic twins.[8]

Critics have argued since the 1930s that the EEA in behavioral twin studies is not supported by the evidence, since when compared with same-sex DZ pairs, MZ pairs grow up experiencing

- Much more similar treatment by parents and others, including being dressed alike;
- More similar physical and social environments, including spending more time together, attending classes together, and having common friends and peer groups;
- More similar treatment by society due to their sharing a very similar physical appearance;
- A greater tendency to model their behavior on each other;
- Identity confusion and a much stronger level of emotional attachment to each other.

By the late 1960s, many twin researchers conceded the point that MZ environments are more similar. In 1978, behavioral geneticist John Loehlin acknowledged that in his 1976 study, he "found, as nearly everybody else has found who has investigated the point, that identical twins are indeed treated more alike — they are dressed alike more often, are more often together at school, play together more, and so forth."[9] A year later, twin researchers Sandra Scarr and Louise Carter–Saltzman concluded that "the evidence of greater environmental similarity for MZ than DZ twins is overwhelming."[10]

More recently, in their 2014 article ironically written in defense of twin research, Barnes and colleagues recognized,

> Critics of twin research have correctly pointed out that MZ twins tend to have more environments in common relative to DZ twins, including parental treatment...closeness with one another...belonging to the same peer networks...being enrolled in the same classes...and being dressed similarly.[11]

Critics do indeed point to these and other environmental influences shared to a much greater degree by MZ twin pairs.

Identity Confusion and Attachment

While recognizing greater MZ versus DZ environmental similarity, twin researchers and their supporters often overlook MZs' much greater levels of attachment, conscious attempts to be alike, and identity confusion. These important points were raised by psychiatrist Don Jackson in his groundbreaking 1960 analysis of schizophrenia genetic research.[12] In *The Trouble with Twin Studies* I presented a table showing the results of all studies I was aware of that assessed levels of twins' identity confusion and psychological attachment to each other. Far from being "equal," most studies found much higher levels of identity confusion and attachment among MZ pairs than among DZ pairs.[13] These findings argue strongly against the EEA's validity because we would expect higher levels of identity confusion and attachment to produce greater MZ behavioral similarity for non-genetic reasons.

Consensus: MZ and DZ Environments Are Different

Twin researchers and their critics don't have to argue anymore about whether MZ and DZ environments are equal, since almost everyone now agrees they are *un*equal. Nevertheless, twin researchers continue to argue that the EEA is valid based on one or more of the eight arguments I describe and analyze below.

Both sides of the EEA debate predict that a behavioral or psychiatric twin study will produce a finding of $rMZ > rDZ$. *The controversy centers on how we should interpret $rMZ > rDZ$.* Behavioral twin researchers and the popularizers of their work argue in favor of a genetic interpretation. Critics, on the other hand, reject the validity of the EEA, and usually argue (1) that $rMZ > rDZ$ can be explained entirely by non-genetic factors, (2) that $rMZ > rDZ$ is uninterpretable, or (3) that twin-method-derived heritability estimates are inflated.

The Model-Fitting Technique

The EEA critique/analysis applies to typical MZ-DZ comparisons, as well as modern twin studies based on the more sophisticated *biometrical model-fitting* technique, which was developed in the 1970s.[14] Researchers using this technique attempt to identify sources of behavioral variation using the "ACE" model, which they believe partitions (A) additive genetic effects, (C) shared family environment, and (E) unique (unshared) environment. Heritability estimates are based on "A." The EEA is seen in "C," where researchers assume that MZ and DZ shared-family environments do not differ. Model-fitting assumptions have been challenged by critics for decades.[15] Whether using simple MZ-DZ comparisons or model-fitting techniques, genetic interpretations of behavioral twin studies are based on accepting the EEA as valid.

Eight Arguments in Defense of the EEA

Faced with the reality of unequal MZ and DZ environments, since the 1950s twin researchers have attempted to sidestep the twin method's unequal environments problem by using one or more of the eight arguments seen in Table 4.2.

In schizophrenia twin research, *Argument A*, *Argument B*, and *Argument H* are the most common ways the EEA has been defended.

I will briefly review these arguments and the main problems found in each. This will be followed by a brief discussion of a 2015 twin study meta-analysis, followed by a critical review of the "EEA-test" study literature.

Argument A: *"Twins create more similar environments for themselves because they are more similar genetically."*

Although twin researchers using *Argument A* recognize that MZs grow up experiencing more similar environments than DZs, they insist that the EEA is valid because MZ pairs, due to their more similar genetically caused behavioral similarities, "create" or "elicit" more similar environments and parental treatment for themselves. Therefore, environmental influences on twins' childhood behavioral similarity should be counted as *genetic* influences. It's as if children create, rather than endure, their own abusive, impoverished,

Table 4.2 Eight Arguments Used by Twin Researchers and Others in Defense of the Equal Environment Assumption

A)	"Twins create more similar environments for themselves because they are more similar genetically. Therefore, environmental influences on twins' childhood behavioral similarity should be counted as genetic influences."
B)	"MZ and DZ environments must be shown to differ on trait-relevant dimensions."
C)	"Assumption violations cancel each other out in favor of heritability."
D)	"MZ behavioral correlations are similar whether twins are reared together or apart."
E)	"The validity of the EEA can be demonstrated mathematically."
F)	"Factors causing MZ behavioral similarities and differences might cancel each other out in favor of genetics."
G)	"The validity of the twin method should be assessed in the context of converging evidence from other types of research."
H)	"Violations of the EEA do not invalidate the twin method, but lead only to inflated heritability estimates."

racist, drug-addicted or alcoholic parent, psychologically cold and distant, and neglectful environments.

An example of *Argument A* is found in a 2000 article by genetic researchers David Evans and Nicholas Martin, writing in support of the "validity of twin studies." Although they recognized that "there is overwhelming evidence that MZ twins are treated more similarly than their DZ counterparts,"

> the more similar parental treatment of MZ vs. DZ twins occurs *in response to* the greater similarity of actions initiated by MZ pairs....It seems...likely that the increased similarity in treatment of MZ twins is a consequence of their genetic identity and the more similar responses this elicits from the environment.[16]

This statement is consistent with Kendler's 1987 argument that studies designed to test the EEA (discussed below) "suggest that the environmental similarity of MZ twins is the *result* and not the cause of their behavioral similarity."[17] Many more examples of *Argument A*, dating back to 1954, can be found in Appendix C of *The Trouble with Twin Studies*.

Supporters of *Argument A* reason that genetic factors explain rMZ > rDZ based on a premise that assumes the very same thing—*a premise based largely on genetic interpretations of previous twin studies*. Twin researchers making use of *Argument A* refer to the genetic premise in support of the genetic conclusion, and then refer back to the genetic conclusion in support of the genetic premise, in a circular loop of faulty reasoning.[18] In other words, they use the twin method to validate the twin method. *Argument A* fails because it is a "heads I win, tails you lose" illogical argument that twin researchers cannot lose, because they count environmental and treatment influences causing greater MZ behavioral similarity as genetic influences.

Argument B: *"MZ and DZ environments must be shown to differ on trait-relevant dimensions."*

Twin researchers using *Argument B* also recognize greater MZ environmental and treatment similarity, but argue that the EEA remains valid until critics are able to identify "trait-relevant" aspects of the environment that cause MZ pairs to behave more similarly. An example of *Argument B* is found in a 1993 publication by Kendler and colleagues:

> The traditional twin method, as well as more recent biometrical models for twin analysis, are predicated on the equal-environment assumption (EEA)—that monozygotic (MZ) and dizygotic (DZ) twins are equally correlated for their exposure to environmental influences *that are of etiologic relevance to the trait under study* [italics added].[19]

It appears that *Argument B* was first used by Irving Gottesman in a 1966 personality twin study. Gottesman redefined the traditional definition of the EEA by inserting one italicized qualifying term into it, now defining the EEA as the assumption "that the average intrapair differences in *trait-relevant* environmental factors are substantially the same for both MZ and DZ twins."[20] This allowed twin researchers to bypass the obviously false EEA as it had been defined since the 1920s, and to place the burden of proof onto critics to show that MZ and DZ environments differ in trait-relevant aspects.

An example of supporters of *Argument B* explicitly shifting the burden of proof from themselves onto critics is seen in Michael Lyons, Kendler, and colleagues' 1991 argument that "it would seem that the burden of proof rests with critics of the twin method to demonstrate that 'trait-relevant' environmental factors are more similar for identical than same-sex fraternal twins."[21] Another example is found in David Rosenthal's 1970 statement that although it is possible that "a higher concordance rate in MZ than DZ twins" is caused by environmental influences, "it must be proved."[22]

A basic principle of science, however, is that the burden of proof falls squarely on the people making a claim, not on their critics. Therefore, given that they recognize that MZ and DZ environments are different, behavioral twin researchers using *Argument B*—and not their critics—are required to identify the *specific and exclusive* trait-relevant environmental factors involved in the behavioral characteristic or psychiatric disorder in question. After identifying such factors, they then must show (1) that MZ and DZ twins did not experience these factors, or (2) that MZ and DZ twins experienced these factors to roughly the same degree. Until they are able to do so, *Argument B* defenses of the EEA fail completely.

Argument C: *"Assumption violations cancel each other out in favor of heritability."*

A third *Argument C* defense of the EEA is that violations of the "random mating" assumption (Assumption 6 in Table 4.1; sometimes called the "no assortative mating assumption"), and violations of the EEA, roughly cancel each other out in favor of genetics and "heritability." Supporters of *Argument C* claim that, whereas unequal MZ and DZ environments might lead to an *over*estimation of heritability, the existence of non-random mating patterns among the biological parents of twins leads to an *under*estimation of heritability. Non-random (assortative) mating is usually defined as the tendency for people to choose mates who are more similar to each other in characteristics ("phenotypes") than would be expected by chance. *Argument C* was a major aspect of Barnes and colleagues' 2014 failed defense of behavioral twin research, and was taken up in 2020 by IQ-hereditarian author Charles Murray, who "summed up" the argument as follows:

> Twin studies have come under criticism for overstating the role of genes. The reality is that violations of the random mating assumption are common

and lead to modest understatement of the role of genes, whereas violations of the equal environments assumption have even more modest effects in the other direction and are uncommon. Overall, heritability as estimated by twin studies appears to be accurate, with errors tending on net to slightly underestimate heritability rather than overestimate it.[23]

To identify the main problem with this argument, let's suppose that the "environmental null hypothesis"—which states that genes that directly cause human behavioral differences do not exist—is true. In this case, mating patterns would have no direct genetic influence on human behavior, and *r*MZ > *r*DZ would be completely caused by non-genetic factors. The contention that non-random mating patterns lead to a "*modest under-statement of the role of genes*" *assumes in advance* that the environmental null hypothesis is false. A twin study, however, is an experiment designed to test *whether* the environmental null hypothesis is false. The findings of this experiment cannot be based on a built-in assumption that it is false, especially since this assumption, once again, is based largely on genetic interpretations of previous twin studies.

Argument D: *"MZ behavioral correlations are similar whether twins are reared together or apart."*

Argument D is based on the results of the tiny handful of TRA (twins reared apart) studies investigating characteristics such as IQ and personality, and the claim that MZ pairs behave similarly regardless of whether they were reared together or reared apart. However, the argument does not take into account the numerous *non-familial* environmental factors and cohort influences that reared-together and reared-apart MZ twins both experience.[24]

TRA studies contain other major flaws and biases, and most MZ pairs found in these studies were only *partially* reared apart.[25] In the most famous study, the Minnesota Study of Twins Reared Apart, the researchers used QRPs to arrive at their conclusions.[26] For these reasons, and also because a technique, test, or research method must stand or fall on its own logic (see *Argument G* below), TRA study results cannot be used to validate genetic interpretations of *r*MZ > *r*DZ.

Argument E: *"The validity of the EEA can be demonstrated mathematically."*

Barnes and colleagues argued in 2014 that the EEA can be validated mathematically by using computer simulations, simulated data, and algebra:

> We have shown empirically that violations of the assumptions of behavioral genetics studies do not invalidate heritability estimates. This is not a matter of opinion but a matter of mathematical evidence.[27]

"There is no room for subjective opinion .... .There is only algebra," they wrote in a subsequent article.[28]

The EEA debate has nothing to do with "algebra," and has everything to do with twins' actual lives, experiences, and development. This includes their childhood and adult social and family environments, and the levels of identity confusion and attachment they experience.

Argument F: *"Factors causing MZ behavioral similarities and differences might cancel each other out in favor of genetics."*

Twin researchers occasionally argue that the environmental similarity of the MZ twinship might lead such pairs to differ from one another, implying that similarity biases and differentiating biases might cancel each other out.[29] Although "reverse biases" in twin research may exist, biases in the direction of creating more behaviorally similar twin pairs are massively larger.

Argument G: *"The validity of the twin method should be assessed in the context of converging evidence from other types of research."*

According to psychologist Scott Lilienfeld and colleagues, pseudoscience proponents "typically maintain that scientific claims can be evaluated only within the context of broader claims and therefore cannot be judged in isolation." As an example, they cited claims by supporters of the Rorschach Inkblot Test that the test should be interpreted in the context of other pieces of information.[30] A version of the "converging evidence" argument was employed by Barnes et al. in 2014, and is seen in this passage from leading psychiatric genetic researchers Stephen Faraone, Ming Tsuang, and a colleague:

> Any conclusion about the role of genes and environment must rely not on a single study or class of study but on the converging evidence provided by a variety of research paradigms.[31]

The validity of the EEA, however, must stand or fall on its own logic, and other sources of "converging evidence" contain their own set of problems. This is also true for the molecular genetic studies and methods I explored in Chapter 2. The twin method cannot be rescued by supposed findings from other research methods when its own key assumption fails.

Argument H: *"Violations of the EEA do not invalidate the twin method, but merely lead to inflated heritability estimates."*

An example of *Argument H* is found in *Behavioral Genetics*, a textbook authored by Robert Plomin and colleagues:

> If the assumption [EEA] were violated because identical twins experience more similar environmental than fraternal twins, this violation would inflate [heritability] estimates of genetic influence.[32]

In *Blueprint*, Plomin avoided the EEA question altogether, even though much of the argument in this 2018 book was based on twin studies. Twin researchers and others using *Argument H* believe that discovering "violations of the EEA" in a particular twin study indicates only that the heritability estimate is inflated, when the proper conclusion is that, due to environmental confounding, the study cannot be interpreted genetically.

Like the first seven arguments, *Argument H* fails to support the EEA, and the only remaining relevant question in assessing the EEA is whether—not why—MZ and DZ environments are different.

A 2015 Twin Study Meta-Analysis

In 2015, behavioral geneticist Tinca Polderman and colleagues published a meta-analysis (analysis of combined studies) based on 2,748 previously published twin studies.[33] The authors of this frequently cited study calculated heritability estimates, based on MZ-DZ correlational differences, for more than 17,000 physical, medical, and psychological characteristics (traits). Remarkably, they did not mention the EEA or cite any evidence that MZ and DZ environments are similar.

If the EEA is false, it doesn't matter whether researchers pool together the results of 5 twin studies, 500 twin studies, or 2,748 twin studies. If the individual behavioral twin studies cannot be interpreted genetically, the pooled results cannot be interpreted genetically either. This meta-analysis merely repeated, on a grand scale, the same interpretive error found in every individual behavioral twin study it counted.

As the British medical statistician Lancelot Hogben warned long ago, almost as if he had the Polderman study in mind, "There is a danger of concealing assumptions which have no factual basis behind an impressive façade of flawless algebra."[34] Due to advances in technology since 1933, we could update Hogben's warning by tacking on the phrase "... and computer-generated online or pdf color graphics, diagrams, and statistical analyses."

The "EEA-Test" Studies

When challenged to defend genetic interpretations of rMZ > rDZ, twin researchers and their supporters usually point to a series of "EEA-test" studies that have appeared since the late 1960s.[35] In these studies, researchers "tested" the validity of the assumption in ways *other* than the only way it can be tested, which is a straightforward determination of whether MZs and same-sex DZs grow up experiencing roughly equal environments—yes or no? If the answer is no, the EEA is false, and genetic interpretations of rMZ > rDZ are wrong. It's that simple.

Ironically, the starting point of most EEA-test publications is a recognition that MZ and DZ childhood environments are *not* equal, as researchers confirmed that MZ twins more often shared the same bedroom growing up, had common friends, were dressed alike, attended school together, and so on. In most cases, however, these researchers concluded that MZ pairs' greater environmental similarity did not constitute a major bias in twin studies, usually by employing one or more of the eight previously discussed arguments.

Four Major Problem Areas

Reviewing over 50 years of EEA-test studies would be as tedious for me to write about (again) as it would be for most people to read. Those interested should consult Chapter 9 of *The Missing Gene*, and a 1996 article by psychologist Alvin Pam and colleagues.[36]

Instead, I will address four problem areas in the EEA-test study literature. These problems also apply to the more recent EEA-test studies I will briefly discuss, by Dalton Conley and colleagues, Jacob Felson, Nancy Segal and colleagues, and Liang-Dar Hwang and colleagues.[37] In general, EEA-test researchers

1. Conducted studies that were subject to problems identified in the replication crisis;
2. Arbitrarily evaluated family studies and twin studies very differently, even though both types of studies compare groups experiencing differing environments;
3. Assumed or implied that most psychiatric genetic and behavioral genetic assumptions, methods, techniques, and diagnoses are valid and largely unchallenged, when in fact they are controversial;
4. Focused narrowly on selected comparisons, while overlooking the larger picture suggesting that $rMZ > rDZ$ cannot be interpreted genetically.

Problem #1: EEA-test Studies Were Subject to Problems Identified in the Replication Crisis

We saw in Chapter 1 that science is in the midst of a replication crisis and that the use of questionable research practices has been rampant for decades, or even from the beginning of behavioral research. We saw that a system allowing people to collect data and analyze results behind the scenes, and to then present their manuscript for publication in an academic journal, is an open invitation to engage in QRPs.

The EEA-test studies were produced by this flawed system, and EEA-test authors had the hidden flexibility to produce any kind of results they wanted. In most cases the people performing these tests had confirmation biases in the EEA-validating direction, and their studies were as vulnerable to p-hacking as any other type of behavioral study.

The 2013 EEA-test study by sociologist Dalton Conley and colleagues used the "misclassified twins" method of testing the EEA, and concluded in favor of "the validity of the equal environment assumption."[38] Like other EEA-test studies, the hidden flexibility problem in non-preregistered behavioral research means that we have no way of knowing, after reviewing the data, whether they conducted and described their study as originally planned, based on their original hypotheses. In his 2017 book *The Genome Factor*, Conley defended the twin method and the EEA based on *Argument A* and *Argument C*.[39]

Most EEA-test studies were performed by twin researchers hoping to validate the EEA (though not Conley's study, according to his account in *The Genome Factor*). Can we really expect them to conclude in favor of the abandonment and invalidation of their life's work? Because the EEA-test studies were not preregistered, we must evaluate them with the same degree of caution as we should evaluate all non-preregistered behavioral studies, if not more.

Problem #2: Arbitrarily Different Evaluations of Family Studies and Twin Studies

Although genetic researchers could use modified versions of *Arguments A–H* in support of interpreting *family study* data in support of genetics, they instead choose to recognize that "family studies by themselves cannot disentangle genetic and environmental influences."[40] This is correct, but because MZ and DZ environments are different, *the same conclusion holds true for twin studies*. EEA-test study authors conceptualize family studies and twin studies as completely different phenomena, when in fact both are kinship studies with similar problems of environmental confounding.

Problem #3: Acceptance of Controversial Psychometric, Psychiatric Genetic, and Behavioral Genetic Assumptions and Methods

Most EEA-test researchers, including Conley, Felson, Segal, and Hwang accept as valid psychometric, psychiatric genetic, and behavioral genetic assumptions, concepts, and methods, even though most are controversial. These include heritability estimates, model-fitting techniques, "general intelligence" or IQ, "personality," and "schizophrenia." We have seen that the reliability and validity of psychiatric diagnoses such as schizophrenia have been challenged by critics. Even Plomin believed that we will have to "tear up our diagnostic manuals based on symptoms," because "there are no disorders to diagnose and there are no disorders to cure."[41]

Problem #4: Narrow Focus on Selected Comparisons

Looking at the larger picture of the results, if we evaluate all behavioral twin studies ever done and take note of the trends, they constitute the grandest EEA-test study of them all. These studies have consistently shown that twin pairs experiencing similar environments and high levels of attachment and identity confusion—MZs—behave much more alike than do pairs experiencing less similar environments and much lower levels of attachment and identity confusion—DZs. A reasonable interpretation of *this* EEA-test study is that $rMZ > rDZ$ can be explained on environmental (non-genetic) grounds.

Lilienfeld and colleagues observed that pseudoscience promoters, "tend to seek only confirming evidence for their claims... . a determined advocate can find at least some supportive evidence for virtually any claim... ."[42] EEA-test researchers answer only questions they choose to ask, and don't "test" or think about the EEA in ways that could suggest that the assumption is false. For example, twin studies of "dog ownership" and "vegetarianism" were conducted for the purpose of calculating heritability estimates for these behaviors.[43] However, the results could easily be transformed into an EEA-test study asking the question: Would a twin study based on an agreed-upon environmentally caused behavior produce a finding of $rMZ > rDZ$? I cannot think of a human behavior less "genetic" than the behavior of choosing not to eat meat when it is available and affordable (vegetarianism/veganism), yet the authors of a twin study concluded that "abstention from meat (i.e., vegetarianism/veganism) was 75% heritable," higher than the 51–57 percent dog ownership heritability estimate, and only slightly lower than current schizophrenia heritability estimates!

Segal and Colleagues' Study

In Segal and colleagues' 2018 study based on "genetically unrelated look-alike" pairs, the authors arrived at the astonishing conclusion that "appearance is not meaningfully related to personality similarity and social relatedness."[44] I say astonishing because, most often, common sense plus research from other fields provide a much better guide to understanding human beings and human development than provided by narrowly focused behavioral genetic "findings" and "laws." "It is quite striking," wrote child psychiatrist Michael Rutter (1933–2021), "that behavioral genetics reviews usually totally ignore the findings on environmental influences. It is almost as if research by non-geneticists is irrelevant."[45]

Segal's study is flawed on numerous grounds, and at best eliminates only one of many environmental factors contributing to MZ twin behavioral resemblance. The researchers' conclusion in favor of genetic influences on personality and self-esteem did not follow from their results.

The Augmented Classical Twin Design

An EEA-test study was published by Liang-Dar Hwang and colleagues in 2021, who developed what they called the "augmented classical twin design" as a way of testing the EEA. To their credit, they recognized that their proposed method was based on "strong assumptions…which may not hold in reality"[46] and recommended the use of "extreme caution" when "applying and interpreting" their method.[47] To the extent that in the future academic journals will continue to publish studies using the twin method, a similar disclaimer should appear at the top of every published behavioral twin study, including the schizophrenia twin studies I will examine in the next chapter.

Summary and Conclusions

I began this chapter with a description of the classical twin method comparison of reared-together MZ and DZ twin pairs, and I emphasized the importance of the twin method's MZ-DZ equal environment assumption (EEA). Although there is widespread agreement that MZ pairs grow up experiencing much more similar environments than DZs, twin researchers and their supporters use various arguments in attempts to support the EEA's validity. I looked at each of these arguments and showed that none supports the EEA. After briefly reviewing a widely cited twin study meta-analysis, I evaluated the "EEA-test study" literature.

There seems to be no end to far-fetched and even comical "findings" from twin method MZ-DZ comparisons, which use the same method employed in the schizophrenia twin studies I will review in the next chapter. Among these we find (in addition to the twin studies of "dog ownership" and vegetarianism) a twin study whose authors concluded in favor of a genetic basis for being a "born again Christian,"[48] a twin study that found important genetic influences on tea and coffee drinking preferences,[49] a twin study that found that the heritability of "loneliness in adults" is 48 percent,[50] a twin study that found genetic influences on "problematic masturbatory behavior,"[51] a twin study that found a moderate genetic aspect of political orientation,[52] and a twin study of "people's desire to be in nature."[53]

MZ pairs behave much more similarly than DZ pairs for just about everything. Twin researchers and their critics agree on this point. The key question is what causes this to occur, and I am not aware of any valid argument in favor of a genetic interpretation of $rMZ > rDZ$ in studies of human behavior. As political scientist Evan Charney concluded in 2013, "That twin studies generate results that even partisans of the methodology acknowledge as absurd is further evidence that they are to many what they have always seemed to be: an obviously confounded, unreliable methodology." [54]

Barnes and colleagues argued against rejecting the twin method. "Scholars should not abandon research or research methods" they wrote. "Instead, they should work to revise their methodologies and statistical models to address known problems."[55] But once environmental confounding in family studies was widely recognized, most genetic researchers eventually *did* abandon genetic interpretations of family study data. Because the EEA is false, we must abandon genetic interpretations of psychiatric and behavioral twin studies as well. In simple language, if the twin method is no good, it's appropriate and necessary to junk it. This conclusion, of course, has major implications for the body of schizophrenia twin research I will examine in the next chapter.

Notes

1 For example, Joseph, J. (1998), The Equal Environment Assumption of the Classical Twin Method: A Critical Analysis, *Journal of Mind and Behavior, 19,* 325–358; Joseph, J. (2002), Twin Studies in Psychiatry and Psychology: Science or Pseudoscience?, *Psychiatric Quarterly, 73,* 71–82. https://doi.org/10.1023/a:1012896802713; Joseph, J. (2004), *The Gene Illusion: Genetic Research in Psychiatry and Psychology under the Microscope*, New York: Algora; Joseph, J. (2006), *The Missing Gene: Psychiatry, Heredity, and the Fruitless Search for Genes*, New York: Algora; Joseph, J. (2015), *The Trouble with Twin Studies: A Reassessment of Twin Research in the Social and Behavioral Sciences*, New York: Routledge.

2 Charney, E. (2012), Behavior Genetics and Postgenomics, *Behavioral and Brain Sciences, 35,* 331–358. https://doi.org/10.1017/S0140525X11002226; Jonsson et al. (2021), Differences Between Germline Genomes of Monozygotic Twins, *Nature Genetics 53,* 27–34. https://doi.org/10.1038/s41588-020-00755-1

3 Alford, J. R., Funk, C. L., & Hibbing, J. R. (2005), Are Political Orientations Genetically Transmitted?, *American Political Science Review, 99,* 153–167, p. 155. https://doi.org/10.1017/S0003055405051579

4 Barnes et al. (2014), Demonstrating the Validity of Twin Research in Criminology, *Criminology, 52,* 588–626, pp. 590, 603. https://onlinelibrary.wiley.com/doi/abs/10.1111/1745-9125.12049

5 Burt, C. H., & Simons, R. L. (2014), Pulling Back the Curtain on Heritability Studies: Biosocial Criminology in the Postgenomic Era, *Criminology, 52,* 223–262. https://doi.org/10.1111/1745-9125.12060; Joseph et al. (2015), The Twin Research Debate in American Criminology, *Logos, 14*(2–3), note 40. http://logosjournal.com/2015/joseph-twin-research/

6 Siemens, H. W. (1924), *Die Zwillingspathologie [Twin Pathology]*, Berlin: Springer Verlag.

7 Newman, H. H., Freeman, F. N., & Holzinger, K. J. (1937), *Twins: A Study of Heredity and Environment*, Chicago, University of Chicago Press, p. 21.

8 Kringlen, E. (1967), *Heredity and Environment in the Functional Psychoses: An Epidemiological-Clinical Study*, Oslo: Universitetsforlaget, p. 20.

9 Loehlin, J. C. (1978), Indentical Twins Reared Apart and Other Routes to the Same Direction, in W. Nance, G. Allen, & P. Parisi (Eds.), *Twin Research, Part A: Psychology and Methodology* (pp. 69–77), New York: Liss, p. 72.

10 Scarr, S., & Carter-Saltzman, L. (1979), Twin Method: Defense of a Critical Assumption, *Behavior Genetics, 9,* 527–542, p. 528. https://doi.org/10.1007/BF01067349

11 Barnes et al., 2014, p. 597.

12 Jackson, D. D. (1960), A Critique of the Literature on the Genetics of Schizophrenia, in D. Jackson (Ed.), *The Etiology of Schizophrenia* (pp. 37–87), New York: Basic Books.

13 Joseph, 2015, pp.166–167. References for the studies in that book's Table 7.1 are listed in the book's reference section.

14 Jinks, J. L., & Fulker, D. W. (1970), Comparison of the Biometrical Genetic, MAVA, and Classical Approaches to the Analysis of Human Behavior, *Psychological Bulletin, 73*, 311–349. https://doi.org/10.1037/h0029135

15 Burt, C. H., & Simons, R. L. (2015), Heritability Studies in the Postgenomic Era: The Fatal Flaw is Conceptual, *Criminology, 53*, 103–112. https://doi.org /10.1111/1745-9125.12060; Goldberger, A. S. (1979), Heritability, *Economica, 46*, 327–347. https://doi.org/10.2307/2553675; Lewontin, R. C. (1974), The Analysis of Variance and the Analysis of Causes, *American Journal of Human Genetics, 26*, 400–411. https://doi.org/10.1093/ije/dyl062T; Taylor, H. F. (1980), *The IQ Game: A Methodological Inquiry into the Heredity-Environment Controversy*, New Brunswick, NJ: Rutgers University Press.

16 Evans, D. M., & Martin, N. G. (2000), The Validity of Twin Research, *GeneScreen, 1*, 77–79, pp. 77–78. https://doi.org/10.1046/j.1466-9218.2000.00027.x

17 Kendler, K. S. (1987), The Genetics of Schizophrenia: A Current Perspective, in H. Meltzer (Ed.), *Psychopharmacology: The Third Generation of Progress* (pp. 705–713), New York: Raven Press, p. 706.

18 Joseph, 2013.

19 Kendler, K. S., Neale, M. C., Kessler, R. C., Heath, A. C., & Eaves, L. J. (1993), A Test of the Equal-Environment Assumption in Twin Studies of Psychiatric Illness, *Behavior Genetics, 23*, 21–27, p. 21. https://doi.org/10.1007/BF01067551

20 Gottesman, I. I. (1966), Genetic Variance in Adaptive Personality Traits, *Journal of Child Psychology and Psychiatry, 7*, 199–208, p. 200. https://doi.org/10.1111 /j.1469-7610.1966.tb02246.x

21 Lyons, M. J., Kendler, K. S., Provet, A. G., & Tsuang, M. T. (1991), The Genetics of Schizophrenia, in Tsuang et al., (Eds.), *Genetic Issues in Psychosocial Epidemiology* (pp. 119–152), New Brunswick, NJ: Rutgers University Press, p. 126.

22 Rosenthal, D. (1970), *Genetic Theory and Abnormal Behavior*, New York: McGraw-Hill, p. 45.

23 Murray, C. (2020), *Human Diversity: The Biology of Gender, Race, and Class*, New York: Twelve, p. 217.

24 Joseph, 2015; Joseph, J. (in press), A Reevaluation of the 1990 "Minnesota Study of Twins Reared Apart" IQ Study, *Human Development*. Available online at https://www.karger.com/Article/Pdf/521922

25 Farber, S. L. (1981), *Identical Twins Reared Apart: A Reanalysis*, New York: Basic Books; Kamin, L. J. (1974), *The Science and Politics of I.Q.*, Potomac, MD: Erlbaum; Kamin, L. J., & Goldberger, A. S. (2002), Twin Studies in Behavioral Research: A Skeptical View, *Theoretical Population Biology, 61*, 83–95. https:// doi.org/10.1006/tpbi.2001.1555; Joseph, 2015, in press; Taylor, 1980.

26 Joseph, 2015; Joseph, in press.

27 Barnes et al., 2014, p. 610.

28 Wright et al. (2015), Mathematical Proof is Not Minutiae and Irreducible Complexity is Not a Theory: A Final Response to Burt and Simons and a Call to Criminologists, *Criminology, 53*, 113–120, p. 114. https://doi.org/10.1111/1745 -9125.12059

29 For examples of this argument, see Joseph, J. (2010), Genetic Research in Psychiatry and Psychology: A Critical Overview, in K. Hood, C. Tucker Halpern, G. Greenberg, & R. Lerner (Eds.), *Handbook of Developmental Science, Behavior, and Genetics* (pp. 557–625), Malden, MA: Wiley-Blackwell.

30 Lilienfeld, S. O., Lynn, S. J., & Lohr, J. M. (2003), Science and Pseudoscience in Clinical Psychology: Initial Thoughts, Reflections, and Considerations, in S. Lilienfeld et al., (Eds.), *Science and Pseudoscience in Clinical Psychology* (pp. 1–14), New York: Guilford, p. 9.

31 Faraone, S. V., Tsuang, M. T., & Tsuang, D. W. (1999), *Genetics of Mental Disorders,* New York: Guilford, p. 32, p. 43. The entire sentence was italicized in the original.

32 Plomin et al., 2013, p. 81.

33 Polderman et al. (2015), Meta-Analysis of the Heritability of Human Traits Based on Fifty Years of Twin Studies, *Nature Genetics, 47,* 702–709. https://doi .org/10.1038/ng.3285

34 Hogben, L. (1933), *Nature and Nurture,* London: George Allen & Unwin, p. 12.

35 Scarr, S. (1968), Environmental Bias in Twin Studies, *Eugenics Quarterly, 15,* 34–40. https://doi.org/10.1080/19485565.1968.9987750

36 Joseph, 2006; Pam et al. (1996), The "Equal Environment Assumption" in MZ-DZ Comparisons: An Untenable Premise of Psychiatric Genetics?, *Acta Geneticae Medicae et Gemellologiae (Twin Research), 45,* 349–360. https://doi .org/10.1017/S0001566000000945

37 Conley et al. (2013), Heritability and the Equal Environments Assumption: Evidence from Multiple Samples of Misclassified Twins, *Behavior Genetics, 45,* 415–426. https://doi.org/10.1007/s10519-013-9602-1; Felson, J. (2014), What Can we Learn from Twin Studies? A Comprehensive Evaluation of the Equal Environments Assumption, *Social Science Research, 43,*184–199. https://doi.org/10.1016/j.ssresearch.2013.10.004; Segal et al. (2018), Pairs of Genetically Unrelated Look-Alikes: Further Tests of Personality Similarity and Social Affiliation, *Human Nature, 29,* 402–417. https://doi.org/10.1007/s12110 -018-9326-2; Hwang et al. (2021), The Augmented Classical Twin Design: Incorporating Genome-Wide Identity by Descent Sharing into Twin Studies in Order to Model Violations of the Equal Environments Assumption, *Behavior Genetics, 51,* 223–236. https://doi.org/10.1007/s10519-021-10044-0

38 Conley et al., 2013, p. 415.

39 Conley, D., & Fletcher, J. (2017), *The Genome Factor: What the Social Genomics Revolution Reveals about Ourselves, our History, and the Future,* Princeton, NJ: Princeton University Press.

40 Plomin et al., 2013, p. 191.

41 Plomin, 2018, pp. 68, 165.

42 Lilienfeld et al., 2003, p. 7.

43 Cinar et al. (2021), Sex Differences in the Genetic and Environmental Underpinnings of Meat and Plant Preferences, preprint. https://psyarxiv.com /7mxar/; Fall et al. (2019), Evidence of Large Genetic Influences on Dog Ownership in the Swedish Twin Registry Has Implications for Understanding Domestication and Health Associations, *Scientific Reports, 9*(1), 7554. https:// doi.org/10.1038/s41598-019-44083-9

44 Segal et al., 2018.

45 Rutter, M. (2006), *Genes and Behavior: Nature-Nurture Interplay Explained,* Malden, MA: Blackwell, pp. 11–12.

46 Hwang et al., 2021, p. 223.

47 Hwang et al., 2021, p. 233.

48 Bradshaw, M., & Ellison, C. G. (2008), Do Genetic Factors Influence Religious Life? Findings from a Behavior Genetic Analysis of Twin Siblings, *Journal for the Scientific Study of Religion, 47,* 529–544. https://doi.org/10.1111/j.1468-5906 .2008.00425.x

49 Luciano et al. (2005), The Genetics of Tea and Coffee Drinking and Preference for Source of Caffeine in a Large Community Sample of Australian Twins, *Addiction, 100,* 1510–1517. https://doi.org/10.1111/j.1360-0443.2005.01223.x

50 Boomsma et al. (2005), Genetic and Environmental Contributions to Loneliness in Adults: The Netherlands Twin Register Study, *Behavior Genetics, 35,* 745–752. https://doi.org/10.1007/s10519-005-6040-8

51 Långström et al. 2002, Genetic and Environmental Influences on Problematic Masturbatory Behavior in Children: A Study of Same-Sex Twins, *Archives of Sexual Behavior, 31,* 343–350. https://doi.org/10.1023/a:1016224326301
52 Alford et al., 2005.
53 Chang et al. (2022), People's Desire to Be in Nature and How They Experience It Are Partially Heritable, *PLoS Biology, 20*(2), e3001500. https://doi.org/10.1371/journal.pbio.3001500
54 Charney, E. (2013), Nature and Nurture [Review of the Book *Man is by Nature a Political Animal,* by P. Hatemi & Rose McDermott (Eds.)], *Perspectives on Politics, 11,* 558–561, p. 560, https://doi.org/10.1017/S1537592713000893
55 Barnes et al., 2014, p. 614.

5   Schizophrenia Twin Research

Sociologists Michael Arribas-Ayllon and colleagues explained how the authors of psychiatric genetic gene-finding and review articles fall back on twin studies to justify continuing the search when faced with disappointing results. They described the following sequence of claims found in these articles: "Identifying genes for psychiatric disorders is difficult. This is because psychiatric disorders are complex. However, history shows that psychiatric disorders are heritable."[1] For the authors of these articles, twin studies supply the main evidence that psychiatric disorders are "heritable."

In psychiatric twin research, twin "concordance rates" are presented as a percentage ranging from 0 percent to 100 percent. Twins are *concordant* for a condition when both members of a pair are affected (diagnosed), and *discordant* when only one member is affected. In psychiatry and other areas of medicine, twins are counted using the dichotomous method of "diagnosed" versus "non-diagnosed." In schizophrenia twin research, investigators identify MZ and DZ pairs in which one twin is diagnosed with schizophrenia, and then determine whether their co-twins are similarly diagnosed. They go on to calculate MZ and DZ group concordance rates as described below. Like other twin studies of behavior, in schizophrenia twin research a finding of $rMZ > rDZ$ is expected by all sides of the debate, with the key question being how we should interpret this finding. As explained in the previous chapter, "$rMZ > rDZ$" is defined as a behavioral twin study finding that MZ pairs resemble each other more than same-sex DZ pairs for the behavioral characteristic or psychiatric disorder in question, at a statistically significant level.

The two methods of calculating twin concordance are the *pairwise method* and the *proband method*. Using the pairwise method, if both twins are diagnosed with schizophrenia in 25 out of 100 pairs, pairwise concordance for schizophrenia is 25/100 = 25 percent. The proband method has gained acceptance among some schizophrenia twin researchers.[2] This method yields the probandwise concordance rate, which double counts the number of concordant pairs and adds the number of concordant pairs to the total number of pairs. Using the proband method, if both twins are diagnosed with schizophrenia in 25 out of 100 pairs, probandwise concordance

DOI: 10.4324/9781003293279-5

for schizophrenia is 50/125 = 40 percent. Because the number of concordant pairs is doubled, the proband method always produces higher concordance rates.

Because schizophrenia twin researchers assume that MZ and DZ environments are equal, they interpret a finding of rMZ > rDZ genetically. They calculate heritability by doubling the MZ-DZ concordance rate difference. For example, researchers finding 40 percent MZ versus 10 percent DZ schizophrenia concordance would calculate a heritability estimate of 60 percent (2x rMZ - rDZ). Since the 1980s, schizophrenia heritability also has been estimated using the biometrical model-fitting technique I described briefly in Chapter 4.

It should be emphasized that schizophrenia twin studies are based on comparisons between reared-*together* MZ and DZ pairs, with each pair growing up together in the same family home. Other than a handful of individual cases of MZ pairs that have come to the attention of researchers since the 1920s, which I discuss briefly toward the end of this chapter, there have been no schizophrenia studies using reared-*apart* twin pairs.

Seventeen Schizophrenia Twin Studies

Schizophrenia twin research dates to 1928, when Hans Luxenburger published his German study.[3] The first American study was published by Aaron Rosanoff and colleagues in 1934.[4] The 17 schizophrenia twin studies and their findings are seen in Table 5.1.

Following Irving Gottesman in *Schizophrenia Genesis*, I have divided the sample into the "classical studies" published between 1928 and 1961, and the "contemporary studies" published since 1963. The classical studies more often contained methodological problems that biased the results in favor of higher MZ concordance rates. These problems included inadequate or vague definitions of schizophrenia, the use of non-blinded diagnoses sometimes based on hearsay or sketchy information about unavailable or deceased twins, the use of inaccurate methods of zygosity determination (whether a pair is MZ or DZ), the use of non-representative or small samples, sample populations that were biased in favor of concordance, and inadequate descriptions of the researchers' methods. The contemporary studies obtained samples from twin registers or consecutive hospital admissions, which produce less-biased samples compared with the older method of obtaining twins from psychiatric hospital populations.[5] A well-known example of the latter is Kallmann's large 1946 study, which reported non-age-corrected concordance rates of MZ = 69 percent, DZ = 11 percent, and age-corrected concordance rates of MZ = 86 percent, DZ = 15 percent.[6]

The pooled MZ pairwise concordance rate across the studies seen in Table 5.1 is 36 percent, while the pooled DZ rate is 6 percent. These figures can be compared with the non-twin general population rate of 1 percent or less. Looking at the 11 methodologically superior contemporary studies

Table 5.1 Results of Schizophrenia Twin Studies

Pairwise Concordance Rates[7]

Researcher(s)/year	Country	MZ Pairs			Same-Sex DZ pairs		
		N	C	%	N	C	%
"Classical Studies"							
Luxenburger (1928) [a]	Germany	17	10	59%	13	0	0%
Rosanoff et al. (1934)	USA	41	25	61%	53	7	13%
Essen-Möller (1941/1970) [b]	Sweden	7	2	29%	24	2	8%
Kallmann (1946)	USA	174	120	69%	296	34	11%
Slater (1953)	UK	41	28	68%	61	11	18%
Inouye (1961)	Japan	55	20	36%	17	1	6%
"Contemporary Studies"							
Tienari (1963/1975)	Finland	20	3	15%	42	3	7%
Gottesman & Shields (1966)	UK	24	10	42%	33	3	9%
Kringlen (1967) [c]	Norway	45	12	27%	69	3	4%
Fischer et al. (1969)	Denmark	25	9	36%	45	8	18%
NAS-NRC (1969/1983) [d]	USA	164	30	18%	268	9	3%
Koskenvuo et al. (1984) [e]	Finland	73	8	11%	225	4	2%
Onstad et al. (1991)	Norway	24	8	33%	28	1	4%
Franzek & Beckmann (1998)	Germany	9	6	67%	12	2	17%
Cannon et al. (1998) [f]	Finland	134	40	30%	374	18	5%
Cardno et al. (1999) [g]	UK	42	13	31%	56	5	9%
Hilker et al. (2017)	Denmark	81	12	15%	367	12	3%
POOLED RATES							
"Classical" (1928–1961)		335	205	61%	464	55	12%
"Contemporary" (1963–2017)		641	151	24%	1,519	68	4%
TOTAL		976	356	36%	1,983	123	6%

N = Number of twin pairs; C = Number of concordant twin pairs.

Concordance rates based on the researchers' "strict" definition of schizophrenia; age correction not included. Unless otherwise noted, when two dates are stated, the first indicates the year results were first published, and the second indicates the final publication, whose figures are reported in the table

[a] Reported by Gottesman & Shields (1966); Gottesman, I. I., & Shields, J. (1966), Contributions of Twin Studies to Perspectives on Schizophrenia, in B. Maher (Ed.), *Progress in Experimental Personality Research* (Vol. 3, pp. 1–84), New York: Academic Press.
[b] MZ figures from Essen-Möller, 1970. DZ concordance rate based on 1941 definite cases among co-twins, as reported by Gottesman & Shields; Gottesman & Shields, 1966, Contributions of Twin Studies to Perspectives on Schizophrenia, p. 28.

Table 5.1 (Continued)

[c] Based on a strict diagnosis of schizophrenia; hospitalized and registered cases
[d] National Academy of Sciences-National Research Council. Original report by Pollin et al., 1969; final report by Kendler and Robinette, 1983
[e] The Koskenvuo et al., study is rarely mentioned in textbooks or reviews
[f] Cannon et al. reported probandwise concordance rates of MZ = 46 percent and DZ = 9 percent. Pairwise rates were not reported. Pairwise rates estimated from sample sizes and probandwise rates
[g] Pairwise data supplied by A. Cardno, personal communication 3/19/2010

published since 1963, the pooled rates fall to 24 percent MZ, 4 percent DZ, meaning that in these studies the MZ co-twin of a person diagnosed with schizophrenia is not so diagnosed about 75 percent of the time.

In the only schizophrenia twin study that assessed levels of identity confusion and attachment among twins, in 1967 Kringlen found that 91 percent of the MZ pairs experienced "identity confusion in childhood," which was true for only 10 percent of the DZ twins. MZ pairs were more likely than DZ pairs to have been "considered as alike as two drops of water" (76% vs. 0%), "brought up as a unit" (72% vs. 19%), and "inseparable as children" (73% vs. 19%). Kringlen's "global evaluation of twin closeness" showed that 65 percent of MZ twins experienced an "extremely strong" level of closeness, which was true for only 19 percent of the DZ pairs.[8]

Rosanoff, Essen-Möller, Slater, Tienari, Kringlen, Gottesman and Shields, and Fischer provided case histories for many of the twin pairs they studied.[9] They at times described concordant MZ pairs using phrases such as "they rather shut themselves up together," "never troubled to make separate friends," "no contact with other people," "they seemed to share one illness between them," "were never separated from one another," "longing intensely for her sister's company," "did not like to mix too much with others," "always clung together," "inseparable," "couldn't make a move without the other," and so on.[10] Social isolation, attachment, and identity confusion are common themes in the case histories of concordant MZ twin pairs.[11]

Gottesman and Shields published their British twin study in 1966. They presented their work in a more detailed format in the 1972 book *Schizophrenia and Genetics: A Twin Study Vantage Point*, which included case history information and diagnoses made by a panel of six schizophrenia experts. One purpose of Gottesman and Shields's study was "to find out what the effects would be on the results when care was taken to avoid, or to make provision for, the alleged sources of error and bias in the earlier 'classical' studies conducted before 1953."[12] They controlled for many of these sources of error and bias except for the most controversial, that is, the EEA.

No Valid Evidence that Schizophrenia is Caused by Genetic Factors

Because the validity of the EEA is the all-important question, it is not necessary to examine and analyze each of the studies in Table 5.1. Instead, because the EEA is false, we can simply conclude that *none of the individual study or pooled results seen in Table 5.1 can be interpreted genetically.* Most genetic researchers would endorse this conclusion when viewing a table of schizophrenia *family* study results, and they should reach the same conclusion when viewing a table of schizophrenia twin study results.

In the remaining sections of this chapter, I will first discuss the results of a study that assessed the EEA specifically for schizophrenia and psychosis. I will then look at an often-cited 2003 schizophrenia twin study meta-analysis, as well as the most recent schizophrenia twin study and the low concordance rates it found. I will then review the story of the "Genain Quadruplets," followed by an example of how schizophrenia twin research is misrepresented in popular works by leading authors. I end the chapter with a brief discussion of two other sources of schizophrenia twin data, followed by some additional conclusions.

Fosse and Colleagues' 2015 Schizophrenia-Specific EEA-Test Study

In 2015, my colleagues, Roar Fosse and Ken Richardson, and I published an analysis of the EEA specifically related to schizophrenia twin research.[13] To the best of our knowledge, the EEA had not been directly tested for schizophrenia with measures of child social adversity, which is a potential environmental cause of schizophrenia and psychosis. If both members of an MZ pair experience child social adversity to a greater degree than both members of a DZ pair, this would lend additional support to the position that the EEA is invalid in twin studies of schizophrenia and psychosis.

Using results from previous non-schizophrenia-related twin studies, we assessed whether MZs correlated higher than DZs for the following five potentially "trait-relevant" (*Argument B*) child social adversity categories: (1) sexual abuse, (2) physical abuse/physical maltreatment, (3) emotional abuse and neglect, (4) bullying, and (5) traumatic life events. The 11 relevant studies encompassed over 9,000 twin pairs and provided 24 comparisons of MZ and DZ intraclass correlations for the five social exposure categories. It was not the aim of these 11 studies to compare MZ and DZ correlations for social adversities, nor were their authors attempting to test the validity of the EEA.

We found significantly higher MZ correlations for each social exposure category. The difference remained consistent across gender, study site (country), sample size, whether psychometric instruments were used, whether interviewing was proximate or distal to the exposures, and whether informants were twins or third persons. We concluded that these results suggest that the EEA is invalid for schizophrenia and other conditions where child adversity is a potentially trait-relevant causative factor. Our study was not preregistered, which is a limitation.

Sullivan and Colleagues' 2003 Meta-Analysis

In 2003, Patrick Sullivan, Kenneth Kendler, and Michael Neale published a schizophrenia twin study meta-analysis (analysis of combined studies).[14] This frequently cited publication (over 2,600 citations as of June 2022, according to Google Scholar) is the usual source for the rough 80 percent schizophrenia heritability estimate.

Sullivan and colleagues calculated an 81 percent heritability estimate from 12 of the 17 studies seen in Table 5.1. Based on their original criteria, only four schizophrenia twin studies qualified for inclusion in the meta-analysis. To include more studies, they "relaxed" their inclusion criteria to increase the sample to 12 studies.[15] A lot could be said about their decision to broaden their criteria to include studies where MZ concordance may have been inflated due to bias, but as always, the EEA is the main issue. For most behavioral characteristics, including schizophrenia, there is no doubt that a meta-analysis will find a result of rMZ > rDZ.

They calculated heritability using the ACE model-fitting technique I discussed in Chapter 4. "Common environmental influences [C]," Sullivan and colleagues wrote, "are shared completely by the members of a twin pair regardless of zygosity [MZ or DZ]."[16] They provided no evidence or citations in support of this claim. Sullivan and colleagues discussed "two key limitations" of their analysis, but the validity of the EEA was not one of them. They concluded, "These meta-analytic results from 12 published twin studies of schizophrenia support a view of schizophrenia as a complex trait that results from both genetic and shared environmental etiological influences."[17] However, because the EEA is false, like the individual studies the results of this meta-analysis cannot be interpreted genetically.

Overlooked Findings

Schizophrenia twin study trends difficult to explain on genetic grounds were not addressed by Sullivan and colleagues. The first is that same-sex DZ pairs are more concordant for schizophrenia than are non-twin siblings, even though both share an average 50 percent genetic relationship.[18] A second trend is that in all schizophrenia twin studies compiling such figures, the pooled pairwise concordance rate for *same*-sex DZs is 2–3 times higher than the *opposite*-sex DZ rate (11.3% vs. 4.7%).[19] Because both types of DZ pairs share the same average genetic relationship to each other, and because male and female schizophrenia prevalence rates are similar, genetic theory predicts that same- and opposite-sex DZ schizophrenia concordance rates should be similar. But they are not.

Earlier Twin Researchers and the EEA

Interestingly, several earlier schizophrenia twin researchers believed that environmental factors explain some portion of rMZ > rDZ. As I showed in *The Gene Illusion*, many of them recognized that environmental factors explain part—although in their opinion only part—of higher MZ concordance rates.[20] For example, Kringlen wrote in 1976,

> The total difference in concordance rate between MZ and DZ twins cannot be ascribed to genetic factors only. A series of studies of both normal and abnormal twins show that the environment of the MZ twin pair is more similar than the environment of the DZ twin pair.[21]

Three more examples are seen below.

Erik Essen-Möller:

> Quite obviously, then, the logical evidence furnished by the classical twin method is not unambiguous, as originally believed. A greater concordance in monozygotics must not invariably depend on their genetic identity, since also their environment may have been more similar.[22]

James Shields:

> The total difference in concordance rate between MZ and DZ twins cannot be ascribed to genetic factors only. A series of studies of both normal and abnormal twins show that the environment of the MZ twin pair is more similar than the environment of the DZ twin pair.[23]

William Pollin and Colleagues:

> An hypothesis like "identification" might account for the higher concordance rate in monozygotic twins without implying a higher incidence of schizophrenia in monozygotic twins. ...Because there are not only genetic but also environmental differences between the monozygotic group and the dizygotic group, differences in concordance rates may be explained by environmental as well as by genetic hypotheses.[24]

These twin researchers believed that their studies showed that genetic factors play a role in causing schizophrenia. Yet in their own way, each researcher recognized that the EEA is false.

Rikke Hilker and Colleagues' 2017 Study

The most recent schizophrenia twin study was published by schizophrenia researcher Rikke Hilker and colleagues in 2017. This study was based on twin pairs identified through Danish psychiatric and twin registers. They used a model-fitting procedure to produce a 79 percent heritability estimate, similar to the 2003 Sullivan estimate.

Although most commentators have focused on Hilker and colleagues' 79 percent heritability estimate, the study found a pairwise MZ schizophrenia concordance rate of only 14.8 percent (12/81 pairs; the researchers calculated a 33% probandwise MZ rate.)[25] Pairwise DZ concordance was only 3.3 percent (12/367). In this study, then, when one member of an MZ twin pair was diagnosed with schizophrenia, 85 percent of the time their genetically identical co-twin was not so diagnosed. This might have led Hilker and colleagues to conclude that non-genetic influences play a major role in causing schizophrenia. However, their apparent desire to "mirror previous reports" and to stay consistent with Sullivan's findings led to a 79 percent heritability estimate, as opposed to the 23 percent estimate they could have arrived at by doubling the pairwise MZ-DZ concordance rate difference (2 × 14.8% - 3.3% = 23% heritability).[26]

Hilker and colleagues assumed that the EEA is valid: "MZ and DZ twin pairs are assumed to share their environment to the same extent, but if MZ twins are exposed to more equal environments than DZ twins the heritability can be overestimated."[27] MZ twins certainly *are* "exposed to more equal environments than DZ twins," but we saw in Chapter 4 that the proper conclusion is not that "heritability is overestimated" (*Argument H*), but that the study cannot be interpreted genetically.

* * *

To this point I have argued that the twin method's equal environment assumption is false, and that a finding of rMZ > rDZ cannot be interpreted genetically in any of the 17 schizophrenia twin studies published to date, or in meta-analyses based on these studies. Changing course a bit, I will now explore the story of identical (MZ) quadruplets concordant for schizophrenia, and how the researchers who studied them conceptualized the causes of their diagnoses.

The *Genain Quadruplets*: "A Study In Child Abuse"

David Rosenthal was a leading research psychologist at the U.S. National Institute of Mental Health (NIMH). Before becoming a major figure in the Danish-American schizophrenia adoption studies I will examine in Chapter 6, he was the lead researcher in a study of reared-together identical female quadruplets, all of whom were diagnosed with schizophrenia. Rosenthal edited and contributed to a 600-page 1963 book about the quads and their family, *The Genain Quadruplets: A Study of Heredity and Environment in Schizophrenia*.[28] He was an admirer of the work of earlier psychiatric genetic researchers, such as Franz Kallmann, Eliot Slater, and others who had trained at Rüdin's Munich institute.[29]

The quadruplets, who were born in 1930 and were raised in the Great Depression and World War II eras in a Midwest U.S. town, were brought to the NIMH and were studied there in the 1950s. Their ages at first hospitalization ranged from 22 to 24.[30] In the book, Rosenthal documented, yet downplayed, the extreme abuse and isolation these young women experienced growing up. He used this case to develop and outline his favored theory of schizophrenia's causation. Critical psychiatrist Peter Breggin called the quadruplets' story "a study in child abuse."[31] We will soon discover why.

"Genain" was a NIMH pseudonym meaning "dire birth" or "dreadful gene," indicating that the researchers assumed in advance that the quads' supposed concordance for schizophrenia was the result of bad heredity.[32] The girls were called "Nora," "Iris," Myra," and "Hester," derived from the NIMH acronym. All four were diagnosed with schizophrenia as young adults. Rosenthal presented this intensely studied family as an example of his belief that a genetic predisposition plus environmental factors can lead to a schizophrenia diagnosis. For Rosenthal and his colleagues, this "once in every one in a half billion births"[33] event must have felt like discovering the Rosetta Stone, or coming into possession of a moonrock.[34]

From another perspective, and with some relevance to the *Hidden Valley Road* story I discussed in Chapter 3, we will see that the Genain quads' story is an example of how inescapable extreme long-term child abuse (including sexual abuse), social isolation, attachment to each other, gender concordance, and identity confusion can lead to psychosis later in life. Although examples of severe abuse are found throughout Rosenthal's lengthy case history, he did not provide a summary of this abuse, or see it as a major cause of the quads' psychoses. Breggin provided a synopsis of the quads' abusive history in his 1991 book *Toxic Psychiatry*, as did Patrick Hahn in his 2019 book *Madness and Genetic Determinism*.[35]

I will now quote in rough chronological order passages from *The Genain Quadruplets* describing the quads' upbringing. We will see that they were raised by unstable and abusive parents, and spent their entire childhood in an inescapable prison house of abuse, which included genital mutilation and constant threats of violence and even death.

The Courtship and Marriage of Henry and Gertrude Genain

Henry Genain told Gertrude that "if she did not marry him, neither she nor he would live to marry anyone else." "The threats of killing increased. At one point, he threatened suicide and remained in bed for three weeks to force her to consent." "She did not love him." "He drank a lot."[36] "On their way to get the [marriage] license, she repeated her unwillingness to marry him. He threatened to kill her. She consented."[37] During sex with her husband, Mrs. Genain "put a pillow over her face to prevent his biting her."[38]

Preschool/Elementary School

For the first six years of their lives, the quads shared their small home with a "strange and unpredictable" psychotic paternal grandmother.[39] "Mr.

Genain drank a great deal and was seldom around the house."[40] Mr. Genain had a "series of extramarital affairs." "Mr. Genain shot at his wife once by accident."[41] "Neighbors, classmates, and teachers unanimously agreed that the girls had no social life....They were not permitted to associate with other children. They never had playmates but played alone in their fenced back yard."[42] Mr. Genain: "There are four of them. They don't need anyone" else.[43] When Mr. Genain drank, "he was abusive and readily lost his temper. Myra said he would threaten to shoot someone and that they were very afraid of him at such times." Mr. Genain told his wife, "If you leave me, I will find you wherever you go and I'll kill you."[44] Hester, who was molested by a school janitor at an early age, began masturbating at the age of three. Mrs. Genain "began to watch Hester vigilantly for signs of this 'disgusting' behavior."[45] Later, "Mr. Genain had discovered Hester masturbating and had swabbed Hester's clitoris with carbolic acid." (Actually, Mrs. Genain did this at Mr. Genain's "bidding."[46]) "It was terrifying and my father discussed using a knife. They would whip her."[47] A doctor "decided to circumcise the girls." After the parents signed the consent form, "the doctor used a great deal of force in preparing her for the operation. The hospital records stated that Iris and Hester Genain were admitted for circumcision and release of adhesions about the clitoris due to chronic masturbation."[48] (Elsewhere in the book, Rosenthal referred to this procedure as "castration."[49]) The doctor "said that he would 'fix her now' and would 'cut all the flesh out.'" The doctor "ordered the girls' hands tied to the bed for thirty nights....During this month, the girls were given sedatives to keep them from crying at night."[50]

Junior High School Years

The quads "always dressed two and two alike, but often all four would wear the same outfit."[51] Some classmates were "teasing and tormenting the girls." "When they left for school in the morning, 'we had to just watch them not to get our books knocked out of our hands, and they would call us everything.' This tormenting continued during school hours." "Myra added, 'we had to watch our step every minute in junior high school.'"[52] "Mr. Genain's earlier restrictiveness increased when the girls became adolescents. He now placed great emphasis on the dangers of associating with boys....Mr. Genain did not want people talking to the girls."[53]

High School Years

"In high school, social activities were still highly restricted." The quads "were not permitted to date nor to attend the usual functions such as football games, school dances, or parties." "They stayed together for the most part, seemingly dependent on each other."[54] "Mrs. Genain said that her husband never permitted the girls to have privacy when they were dressing, especially when they were in high school." Myra "said her father had very set ideas, and that if she and her sisters wanted to do something he did not approve of, he 'would start threatening to shoot himself up, to shoot somebody else up or our family or some tragedy.'"[55] "Hester was manifesting symptoms of severe emotional disorder." "Mrs. Genain said that with Hester's increasing nervousness, the other girl seemed to show anxiety about the possibility of their getting sick too."[56] After Hester told her mother about molestations "by the janitor in elementary school, the boys in junior high school, and the teachers in senior high school," Mrs. Genain told her that she "had not done better because of the sexual misdeeds."[57] Myra said her father "would threaten to commit suicide or kill me or other members of the family…[and] that if anyone got killed I would be the cause of it and in the eyes of God would be a sinful creature deserving punishment; that it would also cause me shame."[58]

Post High School Years

"Although Nora, Iris, and Myra occasionally met young men at work, their father continued to forbid them to go out on dates."[59] "Mrs. Genain said that her husband would wake the girls in the morning when they were working and stay in their rooms until they had removed their pajamas and had put on their brassieres and panties." "Nora told her mother that between the ages of nineteen and twenty-one, when she was alone with her father, he would pat her on the buttocks and feel her breasts."[60] Mr. Genain told Nora: "I'm physically ill; you're mentally ill. I have guns and I may use them, and I'll not leave your mother out."[61] "Mr. Genain spoke to Nora about using his gun to 'stop it all if there is any question of mental trouble in the family.'"[62] "Nora was started on electroshock therapy….pain in her head…blurred vision, dizziness, and inability to bear noise."[63] "Nora said she would like to commit suicide."[64] "Iris made an 'attempt' on her father's life around Easter time."[65] "Mrs. Genain said that [Mr. Genain] entered the washroom when Iris was there, pulled up her dress and tried to pull down her panties. He was 'indecently exposed' and tried to force her against the wall."[66] "There was a great deal of emphasis by the parents on the evils of sex; but Mr. Genain insisted on kissing the girls and fondling their breasts and seeing them nude … and punishing Iris and Hester severely for masturbating."[67] "Iris was again hospitalized from January 2 to January 22 … She was given seven shock treatments."[68] "Iris was again hospitalized with the diagnosis of catatonic schizophrenia … . After four shock treatments (making a total of sixty-seven), she was somewhat more at ease and her mood tended to be euphoric."[69]

Rosenthal's Assessment

Rosenthal described the quads' family environment, and recognized that they grew up "literally fenced in" and were "not permitted to seek out other children."[70] They lived in a virtual prison house where the "blinds were drawn, a fence erected, and the guns kept at the ready."[71] Rosenthal believed there was little doubt that Mr. Genain's daughters "wanted his death."[72]

Before going on, we should consider the following question—would Nora, Iris, Myra, and Hester have become "schizophrenic" if they had grown up apart from each other in four separate abuse-free family environments?

The quads' lifelong history of isolation and abuse was not a major factor in how Rosenthal saw the causes of their schizophrenia diagnoses, however, since he had already accepted the psychiatric genetic point of view that their "dreadful genes" played a major role. He used this family as a backdrop for promoting the "diathesis-stress" model of schizophrenia, which holds that "what is inherited is a constitutional predisposition to schizophrenia," which produces schizophrenia when interacting with non-genetic "exogenous factors."[73] In the Genain quads' case, for Rosenthal their combined experiences supplied the "environmental constriction" stress component of the diathesis-stress model. "All things considered," Rosenthal concluded, "this is the model that I think best fits the patterns of illness in the Genain quadruplets."[74]

Rosenthal can be criticized for greatly de-emphasizing the impact of the sexual, mental, physical, medical, and psychiatric abuse these girls had to endure (Iris was electroshocked 67 times), and for downplaying how isolation, attachment, and identity confusion can lead people to exhibit similar behaviors. Mr. Genain, with help from his wife, isolated the girls from an early age and used violence and threats of violence to keep them for himself, in part for his own sexual gratification. As Hahn concluded, "Neither Rosenthal nor any of his co-authors ever ask the obvious question: who wouldn't be crazy after surviving that horror show of a childhood?"[75] A commitment to psychiatric genetic approaches is also a commitment to never ask these types of questions.

In his 2014 book, *The Body Keeps the Score: Brain, Mind, and Body in the Healing of Trauma*, psychiatric trauma researcher Bessel van der Kolk described the famous "learned helplessness" experiments on dogs, in research headed by Martin Seligman and Steven Maier. van der Kolk wrote of the "inescapable shock" experienced by many trauma survivors he had worked with:

> What they had done to these poor dogs was exactly what had happened to my traumatized human patients. They, too, had been exposed to somebody (or something) who had inflicted terrible harm on them— harm they had no way of escaping. I made a rapid mental review of the patients I had treated. Almost all had in some way been trapped or immobilized, unable to take action to stave off the inevitable. Their fight/flight response had been thwarted, and the result was either extreme agitation or collapse.[76]

van der Kolk described environments leading to later trauma symptoms and a diagnosis of post-traumatic stress disorder (PTSD). It's not a stretch to consider the likelihood that, regardless of their genes, the "inescapable terrible harm" inflicted on four socially isolated female siblings during their entire childhood and early adulthood led to their shared "collapse," and to their shared psychosis.

Folie à Deux, Folie à Quatre

Folie à deux (shared psychotic disorder) has been defined as "a psychiatric entity characterized by the transference of delusional ideas and/or abnormal behavior from one person to one or more others who have been in close association with the primarily affected person."[77] In his groundbreaking 1960 critique of schizophrenia genetic research, family systems therapy pioneer Don Jackson addressed the relationship between folie à deux and concordance for schizophrenia among MZ twins.[78] Jackson observed that close attachment and social isolation were often seen in the case histories of concordant MZ twin pairs, especially among female MZ pairs.

In a 1960 article on schizophrenia twin research, Rosenthal weighed in on this issue:

> One could imagine a [MZ] co-twin being drawn toward schizophrenic behavior if his twin had become schizophrenic and if he felt himself to be so much like his twin that he was completely convinced that the fate which had befallen his twin would befall him as well. He might be unable to resist this conviction, and presumably could behave in accordance with it.[79]

Well put, and here Rosenthal characterized schizophrenia as a behavior a person could be "drawn toward," rather than a disease. Yet three years later in *The Genain Quadruplets*, Rosenthal saw heredity and much less important "exogenous factors" as the main explanation for the quads' concordance for schizophrenia, and largely ignored the possibility that they were "unable to resist" similar fates for psychological reasons.

The tragic story of the Genain sisters shows in gruesome detail how psychosis can be "transmitted" through severe abuse, mutilation, constant threats of violence and of being killed, close psychological association, isolation, and identity confusion—in other words, *folie à quatre*.

Later Analyses

The quads were brought to the NIMH for follow-up studies at the ages of 27, 51, and 66. They were administered neuropsychological examinations that included a battery of psychological tests. All four women took neuroleptic ("anti-psychotic") medication. The NIMH researchers attributed potential differences in the quads' brains to possible birth trauma, but apparently not to childhood trauma, the powerful medications they took, or to the fact that at least two had endured numerous electroshock sessions.[80]

As a young intern, Lynn DeLisi managed procedures and helped care for the quads during their two-month stay at the NIMH inpatient ward. In her 2017 book *100 Questions & Answers about Schizophrenia: Painful Minds*, DeLisi described how working with the Genain family left the "deep impression" in her memory that "no family could have such bad luck as to have all four of their children diagnosed with schizophrenia *unless the illness was genetic.*"[81] From another perspective, however, we could say that no quadruplets could have such bad luck as to have been born into a family with Henry and Gertrude Genain as their parents. DeLisi was proud to have received Rosenthal's personal copy of *The Genain Quadruplets*, but her account mentioned nothing about the conditions the sisters were forced to endure while growing up, as if horrifying abuse had little or no relevance to what she viewed as their shared "genetic illness." We have already seen that DeLisi overlooked "torrents" of abuse in the *Hidden Valley Road* Galvin family as well.

Psychologist Nancy Segal wrote a 2001 article about the original Genain study and the follow-up studies. One of the world's most well-known twin researchers, Segal failed to mention the history of severe abuse experienced by the quads, or the fact that they had been mutilated and electroshocked by medical authorities. A great admirer of Rosenthal's work, Segal ended by writing, "I think of David Rosenthal often, and his wonderful research legacy."[82] I too think often of Rosenthal's research legacy, but in the following chapter we will see that my evaluation of his legacy differs radically from Segal's.

Rosenthal's team interviewed people in the Genain family's community of "Envira" (for environment), who had known the family when the girls were growing up. He seemed almost amused that all these non-behavioral-scientist townspeople "volunteered an opinion as to what caused the illness." In "every case but one," said Rosenthal, "the interviewee identified the cause as something the father or mother or both had or had not done in rearing the girls." Only one person in the community thought heredity was involved. That person was a geneticist, "and he, too, said that the parents were too strict with the children!"[83]

There are times when common sense, and a simple "lay" understanding of how people can be psychologically damaged and broken, is superior to the opinions of advanced-degree-holding expert behavioral scientists wedded to genetic theories leading them to overlook, or minimize, the harm people can do to one another. For psychologist Richard Bentall, Rosenthal and his fellow Genain investigators did not emphasize the appalling abuse in that family "because the genetic explanation for schizophrenia seemed to be so self-evidently true that it blinded them to what would have been obvious to anyone else," including, of course, the astute townspeople of Envira.[84]

A Pulitzer Prize Winner Gets the Facts Wrong

In his bestselling 2016 book *The Gene: An Intimate History*, cancer physician and researcher Siddhartha Mukherjee told the "story of the gene" and the history of genetic research and theories, detailing discoveries as well as horrible abuses and crimes committed in the name of genetics and eugenics.[85] Mukherjee weaved his own family history of psychosis and mental disorder into the story. He believed that heredity was a major cause of these conditions, as well as a major influence on human behavioral differences (variation) in general. This was a central conclusion of the book:

> Gender. Sexual preference. Temperament. Personality. Impulsivity. Anxiety. Choice. One by one, the most mystical realms of human experience have become progressively encircled by genes. Aspects of behavior relegated largely or even exclusively to cultures, choices, and environments, or to the unique constructions of self and identity, have turned out to be surprisingly influenced by genes.[86]

There are some interesting areas in Mukherjee's book, including a discussion of twin research having its origins in eugenics and the German racial hygiene movement, an area I covered in more depth in my 2004 book *The Gene Illusion*. Twin researchers and their supporters rarely mention the eugenic origins of their field.[87] Yet Mukherjee's book provides an example of an inaccurate and misleading account of schizophrenia genetic research by a respected author. Previously, Mukherjee won the Pulitzer Prize for his 2011 book *Cancer: The Emperor of All Maladies*.

In *The Gene*, Mukherjee stressed what he saw as the importance of performing "twins reared apart" (TRA) studies because, as he correctly observed, genetic interpretations of MZ twin behavioral resemblance are "intrinsically flawed" because reared-together MZ pairs are treated similarly by parents, teachers, and others. This led to a "conceptual gridlock" in studies of reared-together MZ pairs, Mukherjee wrote, because "geneticists knew" that studying such pairs involved the "*impossibility* [italics added] of unbraiding the twisted strands of nature and nurture."[88] Although comparing reared-together MZs to reared-together DZs "partially solved the problem," he noted that critics argue that MZ-DZ comparisons "were also intrinsically flawed." For Mukherjee, TRA studies were necessary because the twin method had reached an "impasse."[89]

However, in his discussion of the schizophrenia twin studies, Mukherjee seemed to forget all this and claimed that these studies showed that "it was impossible to deny a genetic cause" of schizophrenia.[90]

Schizophrenia Twin and Genetic Research
Did Not Begin in the 1970s

"The first clues about the etiology of schizophrenia," Mukherjee wrote, "came from twin studies. In the 1970s, studies demonstrated a striking degree of concordance among twins." Strangely, Mukherjee cited a 1977 *autism* twin study publication as the single source of his claim, whose authors mentioned schizophrenia twin research only briefly and in relation to autism.[91] The "first clue" schizophrenia twin study did not appear "in the 1970s," but rather in 1928, and ten more were published between 1929 and 1969 (see Table 5.1). In fact, no original-data schizophrenia twin studies were published in the 1970s. Mukherjee said that Irving Gottesman's schizophrenia twin study was published in 1982. The actual publication year was 1966.[92]

Mukherjee discussed the "enormous National Academy of Sciences (NAS) study [that] published [twin] data definitively linking schizophrenia to genetic causes," which used "the twin method pioneered by Galton..."[93] But as we just saw, elsewhere in the book he called such claims into question by recognizing that the twin method had arrived at an "impasse," due to its inability to satisfactorily separate nature and nurture influences. He said that the NAS study found that "identical twins possessed a striking 30 to 40 percent concordance rate for schizophrenia."[94] But there was nothing "striking" about this result, since other researchers had reported similar or higher schizophrenia concordance rates since the 1920s.

The original NAS twin study was published in 1969 by psychiatrist William Pollin and his colleagues, and was based on twins identified through a U.S. Veterans Administration registry.[95] The results that Mukherjee cited were taken from a 1983 update/reanalysis of this study by Kendler and Dennis Robinette, who obtained additional records enabling them to increase the original MZ sample of 69 to 164.[96] The final 1983 NAS study pairwise concordance rate was only 18.3 percent (30/164), but Kendler and Robinette emphasized 30.9 percent MZ concordance by using the proband concordance method.

Pollin and colleagues' original 1969 NAS study pairwise MZ concordance rate was only 13.8 percent (11/69), which led them to conclude that the "role of the suggested genetic factor appears to be a limited one."[97] Hilker and colleagues, on the other hand, found very similar MZ pairwise concordance in 2017 (14.8%, 12/81), yet they concluded that schizophrenia carries a "high genetic risk."[98] Twin research results never speak for themselves. Interpretation is everything.

"Fleets" of Nonexistent 1980s Schizophrenia Twin Studies

According to Mukherjee, "throughout the 1980s, fleets of twin studies strengthened the case for a genetic cause of schizophrenia."[99] In "study upon study," he wrote, "the concordance among identical twins exceeded that of fraternal twins so strikingly that it was impossible to deny a genetic cause." These unreferenced "fleets" of 1980s twin studies, in Mukherjee's view, helped "bring sanity to the study of madness" because they helped overturn unsupported "seductive" psychoanalytic explanations of psychosis.[100]

Apart from the above-mentioned 1983 NAS update, however, only one original-data schizophrenia twin study was published in the 1980s, by Koskenvuo and colleagues in 1984. This study is almost never mentioned by schizophrenia twin researchers, or found in textbooks or in schizophrenia genetics review articles. For the most part, without explanation, the 1984 Koskenvuo et al. twin study does not exist in the mainstream genetics of schizophrenia literature. Similar to Pollin and Hilker, Koskenvuo and colleagues found a very low, 11 percent (8/73), MZ concordance rate.[101]

In the 2003 Sullivan meta-analysis, the only 1980s twin study listed was the Kendler and Robinette study, and the only 1970s twin study listed was Pekka Tienari's final 1975 report based on his original 1963 Finnish study.[102] Regardless of what Mukherjee said, Koskenvuo's little-known 1984 investigation and Kendler and Robinette's NAS update were the only original-data schizophrenia twin studies published between 1970 and 1990. The combined pairwise MZ schizophrenia concordance rate in these two studies was a modest 16 percent (38/237; see Table 5.1).

How Mukherjee was able to conjure up multiple "first clue" 1970s schizophrenia twin studies, followed by additional "fleets" of such studies in the 1980s, I haven't a clue. Although much of what he wrote about schizophrenia twin research was wrong—just as much of what he wrote about the Minnesota Study of Twins Reared Apart was also wrong—Mukherjee's status as a Pulitzer Prize–winning medical authority helps create and perpetuate myths about genetic research.[103]

Ken Burns' Documentary

Mukherjee's book was the subject of a two-part four-hour 2020 U.S. Public Broadcasting System (PBS) documentary by the famous filmmaker Ken Burns, titled "Ken Burns Presents *The Gene: An Intimate History.*" Prior to production, I had been in e-mail communication with a company working on the documentary, and I shared my earlier articles highlighting Mukherjee's major mistakes and lack of knowledge about twin research, upon which the main arguments in his book were based.[104] I think this had an impact.

Burns' four-hour documentary devoted only two minutes to schizophrenia, reporting that "by the 1990s, geneticists knew that schizophrenia often ran in families."[105] They actually "knew" this at least 80 years earlier, when Kraepelin and Bleuler (mistakenly) used this observation to support their beliefs about hereditary causes, and when Rüdin published his 1916 family study. Burns committed the fallacy of assuming that schizophrenia running in the family provides "a powerful clue that it must have a genetic basis." Mukherjee made the same mistake in the book: "Families with well-established histories of schizophrenia and bipolar disease—such as mine—were documented across multiple generations, again demonstrating a genetic cause."[106]

The film portrayed schizophrenia as a genetic disorder, like actual genetic disorders discussed in other parts of the film, such as Huntington's Disease, Spinal Muscular Atrophy (SMA), and the KIF1A-Related Disorder. Of these three conditions, only Huntington's was discussed in the book. Burns utilized mid-20th-century films of bizarrely behaving backward schizophrenia patients to suggest that current schizophrenia patients belong in a category similar to the above-mentioned real genetic disorders. Stacey Gabriel, Chief Genomics Officer of the Broad Institute, acknowledged in the film that earlier molecular genetic studies of schizophrenia "found absolutely no signal." Predictably, Gabriel then said that after greatly increasing the sample sizes, "finally some signals emerged." The narrator said that the findings showed that schizophrenia "genetic mutations were scattered all over the genome." The views of the critics were not presented in Burns' documentary.

Genetic researcher David Goldstein said in the film that although associated regions on the genome have been identified, in "almost none" of the regions "have we actually tracked down to the exact responsible genes" for schizophrenia. The documentary drew no conclusions about this statement, but it did show Goldstein looking uncomfortable when he had to admit, even if understatedly, that from the standpoint of helping create "new therapies [i.e., drugs]. ...Genome-wide association studies have worked *less* well than hoped for."

Twin research was totally absent in the documentary. In the book Mukherjee highlighted the Minnesota Study of Twins Reared Apart as the centerpiece of the idea that aspects of human behavior, once thought to be the result of our environment, "have turned out to be surprisingly influenced by genes." There was no mention of this study in the documentary. Other than schizophrenia, for the most part human behavior was left out of Burns' film, and the conditions discussed were mainly real (non-psychiatric) genetic medical disorders such as those I mentioned above.

I imagine that the planned focus of Burns' documentary was significantly changed from the major themes of the book such as schizophrenia, Mukherjee's family history of "madness," behavioral genetics, and twin studies when Mukherjee was unable to provide a satisfactory answer to Burns and the producers about what I had written in my articles versus what he had written in his book.

Other Schizophrenia Twin Designs

The Offspring of Discordant MZ Pairs Design

Two other types of schizophrenia twin studies should be mentioned. The first studied schizophrenia rates among the biological offspring of *dis*cordant reared-together MZ pairs (one twin is diagnosed with schizophrenia, while the other is not). Psychiatric geneticist Margit Fischer introduced this method into twin research in 1971, after which appeared a frequently cited 1989 follow-up study based on Fischer's pairs by Gottesman and Aksel Bertelsen.[107] Genetic theories predict finding comparable schizophrenia rates among the offspring of these pairs, and this is what these researchers said they found.

However, the design is unable to adequately separate potential genetic and environmental influences, and small samples make it unlikely that statistically significant differences will be found between these offspring groups. The discordant co-twins grew up in the same family, and like most MZ pairs they experienced similar environments and treatments. Most of the environmental factors that could have contributed to a schizophrenia diagnosis in one of the twins were probably also experienced by their "well" co-twin, who could have transmitted psychologically unhealthy rearing patterns toward their offspring. There are also doubts about the accuracy of the diagnoses, especially since most of the offspring were not personally examined by the researchers.[108]

Psychiatrist E. Fuller Torrey considered Fischer's case material to be "markedly unsatisfactory," and found that none of the MZ pairs "met the basic criteria for twins with clearly diagnosed schizophrenia in the index twin and verifiable (i.e., based on interview) normality in the co-twin." Torrey argued that Gottesman and Bertelsen's decisions about which twins to retain or remove were "entirely arbitrary," and that their conclusion in favor of genetic factors "is premature at best."[109] More details on problems with these studies can be found elsewhere, and like all behavioral research we must evaluate Gottesman and Bertelsen's findings in the context of the replication crisis.[110]

Twins Reared Apart

Although no systematic schizophrenia "reared-apart" twin study has ever been performed, there have been a few single-case reports of purportedly reared-apart MZ pairs concordant or discordant for schizophrenia. In psychologist Susan Farber's 1981 review of these cases, she concluded that only nine MZ pairs qualified as having been truly reared-apart.[111] However, even in these cases the twins were aware of each other's existence and had periodic contact. These reports have a built-in bias toward finding concordant pairs because researchers, hospital administrators, and others are more likely to hear about a pair of separated MZ twins hospitalized for schizophrenia, whereas a discordant pair would not come to their attention as often. In addition, for various reasons researchers and journalists might decide against investigating or writing about discordant pairs they hear about.

To mention one reportedly concordant pair I discussed in *The Gene Illusion*, which was originally described by W. H. Craike and Eliot Slater in 1945, Edith and Florence were British MZ twins separated nine months after birth. Florence was adopted by a maternal aunt. Edith stayed with her father until the age of eight, when she was placed in a children's home. They did not meet again until age 24, but each was aware of the other's existence. Edith reported that while living with her father, "Florence was making trouble for her by writing to her father and telling him Edith had told her that he was a drunkard." Edith also believed that Florence was watching her house and had been plotting against her. Their supposed delusional systems were based on mutual distrust. According to Craike and Slater's description,

> each twin occupies for the other an over-valued position; to each the other is supremely important, although the circumstances of their lives touch at few points. Edith at first sight places Florence at the center of her persecutors; Florence, with her own inborn tendency to paranoia, reacts to this by coming in her turn to regard Edith as her chief enemy.[112]

Although Craike and Slater said that Edith and Florence "were brought up along entirely different lines," they recognized that "each sister centers her delusions around the other."[113] This pair provides an example of what Howard Taylor rightly called the "myth" of separated MZ twins in behavioral research.[114]

As the saying goes, "The plural of anecdote is not data." Perhaps this explains why Gottesman concluded in 1982, "After a quarter century of experience with twins reared together and twins reared apart, it is my conviction that twins reared apart are a wonderful source of hypothesis generation, but not a useful source for hypothesis testing."[115]

Summary and Conclusions

The main conclusion I reached in this chapter was built upon the conclusions I reached in the previous chapter. Because the EEA is false, none of the 17 schizophrenia twin studies seen in Table 5.1, or the pooled or meta-analyzed results, can be interpreted genetically. A study my colleagues and I published was designed to test the EEA in schizophrenia twin research. Although our study was not preregistered, our findings provided additional evidence that the assumption is not valid for schizophrenia twin research. I then performed a brief critical review of a schizophrenia twin study meta-analysis, as well as the most recently published twin study. I described the tragic story of the "Genain Quadruplets," and showed how researchers committed to genetic theories can overlook the potentially crazy-making impact of severe abuse experienced by isolated siblings. As an example of the widespread misreporting of genetic research, I showed how Siddhartha Mukherjee described schizophrenia twin research in *The Gene: An Intimate History*, and I reviewed Ken Burns' documentary based on the book. Finally, I described the offspring of discordant MZ pairs design, and the few pairs of supposedly reared-apart MZ twins concordant for schizophrenia. I showed that neither method has supplied evidence in support of genetic causes of schizophrenia and psychosis.

Because the EEA is false, it is likely that twin studies of schizophrenia and psychosis have recorded nothing more than research bias, MZ pairs' more similar environments and treatment, MZ pairs' higher levels of identity confusion and attachment to each other, MZ pairs' greater tendency to model their behavior on each other, and MZ pairs' greater tendency to experience folie à deux (shared psychotic disorder) than DZ pairs. Kendler wrote in a 1993 article, "With some uniformity, the available empirical evidence suggests that the EEA is probably at least approximately correct for the normative traits and psychiatric disorders studied."[116] This single sentence by the leading theoretical defender of psychiatric twin studies contains hedged terms such as "some uniformity," "available empirical evidence," "suggests," "probably," "at least," "approximately," and "normative." It is hardly a ringing endorsement of the EEA.[117]

I have shown in Chapters 4 and 5 that the results of schizophrenia twin research cannot be interpreted genetically, and therefore, like family studies, they provide no evidence in support of genetic theories of schizophrenia. In the next chapter I will examine the final shaky pillar of support for these theories: studies of adopted children and their relatives.

Notes

1 Arribas-Ayllon, M., Bartlett, A., & Lewis, J. (2019), *Psychiatric Genetics; From Hereditary Madness to Big Biology*, London: Routledge, p. 85.
2 McGue M. (1992), When Assessing Twin Concordance, Use the Probandwise Not the Pairwise Rate, *Schizophrenia Bulletin, 18,* 171–176. https://doi.org/10.1093/schbul/18.2.171
3 Luxenburger, H. (1928), Vorläufiger Bericht über Psychiatrische Serienuntersuchungen an Zwillingen [Provisional Report on a Series of Psychiatric Investigations of Twins], *Zeitschrift fur die Gesamte Neurologie und Psychiatrie, 116,* 297–347.
4 Rosanoff et al. (1934), The Etiology of So-Called Schizophrenic Psychoses, *American Journal of Psychiatry, 91,* 247–286. https://doi.org/10.1176/ajp.91.2.247
5 Rosenthal, D. (1970), *Genetic Theory and Abnormal Behavior,* New York: McGraw-Hill.
6 Kallmann, F. J. (1946), The Genetic Theory of Schizophrenia: An Analysis of 691 Schizophrenic Twin Index Families, *American Journal of Psychiatry, 103,* 309–322. https://doi.org/10.1176/ajp.103.3.309
7 Luxenburger, H. (1928), Vorläufiger Bericht über Psychiatrische Serienuntersuchungen an Zwillingen [Provisional Report on a Series of Psychiatric Investigations of Twins], *Zeitschrift fur die Gesamte Neurologie und Psychiatrie, 116,* 297–347; Rosanoff et al. (1934), The Etiology of So-Called Schizophrenic Psychoses, *American Journal of Psychiatry, 91,* 247–286. https://doi.org/10.1176/ajp.91.2.247; Essen-Möller, E. (1941), Psychiatrische Untersuchungen an einer Serie von Zwillingen [Psychiatric investigations on a series of twins], *Acta Psychiatrica et Neurologica* (Suppl. 23), Copenhagen: Munksgaard; Essen-Möller, E. (1970), Twenty-one Psychiatric Cases and

Their MZ Cotwins. *Acta Geneticae Medicae et Gemellologiae, 19,* 315–317. https://doi.org/10.1017/S1120962300025798; Kallmann, F. J. (1946), The Genetic Theory of Schizophrenia: An Analysis of 691 Schizophrenic Twin Index Families, *American Journal of Psychiatry, 103,* 309–322. https://doi.org /10.1176/ajp.103.3.309; Slater, E. (1953), Psychotic and Neurotic Illnesses in Twins, *Medical Research Council Special Report Series No. 278,* London: Her Majesty's Stationary Office; Inouye, E. (1961), Similarity and Dissimilarity of Schizophrenia in Twins, *Proceedings of the Third World Congress of Psychiatry* (Vol. 1, pp. 524–530), Montreal: University of Toronto Press; Tienari, P. (1963), *Psychiatric Illnesses in Identical Twins,* Copenhagen: Munksgaard; Tienari, P. (1975), Schizophrenia in Finnish Male Twins, *British Journal of Psychiatry Special Publication, No. 10,* M. Lader (Ed.), pp. 29–35; Gottesman, I. I., & Shields, J. (1966), Schizophrenia in Twins: 16 Years' Consecutive Admissions to a Psychiatric Clinic, *British Journal of Psychiatry, 112,* 809–818. https://doi .org/10.1192/bjp.112.489.809; Kringlen, E. (1967), *Heredity and Environment in the Functional Psychoses: An Epidemiological-Clinical Study,* Oslo: Universitetsforlaget; Fischer, M., Harvald, B., & Hauge, M. (1969), A Danish Twin Study of Schizophrenia, *British Journal of Psychiatry, 115,* 981–990. https://doi.org/10.1192/bjp.115.526.981; Pollin et al. (1969), Psychopathology in 15,909 Pairs of Veteran Twins: Evidence for a Genetic Factor in the Pathogenesis of Schizophrenia and its Relative Absence in Psychoneurosis, *American Journal of Psychiatry, 126,* 597–610. https://doi.org/10.1176/ajp .126.5.597; Kendler, K. S., & Robinette, C. D. (1983), Schizophrenia in the National Academy of Sciences-National Research Council Twin Registry: A 16-year Update, *American Journal of Psychiatry, 140,* 1551–1563. https:// doi.org/10.1176/ajp.140.12.1551; Koskenvuo et al. (1984), Psychiatric Hospitalization in Twins, *Acta Geneticae Medicae et Gemellologiae, 33,* 321– 332. https://doi.org/10.1017/S0001566000007364; Onstad et al. (1991), Twin Concordance for DSM-III-R Schizophrenia, *Acta Psychiatrica Scandinavica, 83,* 395–401. https://doi.org/10.1111/j.1600-0447.1991.tb05563.x; Franzek, E., & Beckmann, H. (1998), Different Genetic Background of Schizophrenia Spectrum Diagnoses: A Twin Study, *American Journal of Psychiatry, 155,* 76–83. https://doi.org/10.1176/ajp.155.1.76; Cannon et al. (1998). The Genetic Epidemiology of Schizophrenia in a Finnish Twin Cohort, *Archives of General Psychiatry, 55,* 67–74. https://doi.org/10.1001/archpsyc.55.1.67; Cardno et al. (1999), Heritability Estimates for Psychotic Disorders, *Archives of General Psychiatry, 56,* 162–168. https://doi.org/10.1001/archpsyc.56.2.162; Hilker et al. (2017), Heritability of Schizophrenia and Schizophrenia Spectrum Based on the Nationwide Danish Twin Register, *Biological Psychiatry, 83,* 492–498. https://doi.org/10.1016/j.biopsych.2017.08.017

8   Kringlen, E. (1967), *Heredity and Environment in the Functional Psychoses: An Epidemiological-Clinical Study,* Oslo: Universitetsforlaget, p. 115.

9   The Fischer, Gottesman & Shields, and Kringlen case histories can be found in Fischer, M. (1973), *Genetic and Environmental Factors in Schizophrenia,* Copenhagen: Munksgaard; Gottesman, I. I., & Shields, J. (1972), *Schizophrenia and Genetics: A Twin Study Vantage Point,* New York: Academic Press; Kringlen, E. (1967), *Heredity and Environment in the Functional Psychoses: Case Histories,* Oslo: Universitetsforlaget.

10   References for these case history excerpts can be found in Joseph, J. (2004), *The Gene Illusion: Genetic Research in Psychiatry and Psychology Under the Microscope,* New York: Algora, pp. 178–184.

11   Jackson, D. D. (1960), A Critique of the Literature on the Genetics of Schizophrenia, in D. Jackson (Ed.), *The Etiology of Schizophrenia* (pp. 37–87), New York: Basic Books.

12 Gottesman & Shields, 1972, p. xvi.

13 Fosse R., Joseph J., & Richardson, K. (2015), A Critical Assessment of the Equal Environment Assumption of the Twin Method for Schizophrenia, *Frontiers in Psychiatry, 6:62*, 1–10. https://doi.org/10.3389/fpsyt.2015.00062

14 Sullivan, P. F., Kendler, K. S., & Neale, M. C. (2003), Schizophrenia as a Complex Trait: Evidence from a Meta-Analysis of Twin Studies, *Archives of General Psychiatry, 60*, 1187–1192. https://doi.org/10.1001/archpsyc.60.12.1187

15 Sullivan et al., 2003, p. 1188.

16 Sullivan et al., 2003, p. 1188.

17 Sullivan et al., 2003, p. 1191.

18 Joseph, J. (1998), *A Critical Analysis of the Genetic Theory of Schizophrenia*, unpublished doctoral dissertation, California School of Professional Psychology, Alameda; Lewontin, R. C., Rose, S., & Kamin, L. J. (1984), *Not in Our Genes: Biology, Ideology, and Human Nature*, New York: Pantheon.

19 Jackson, 1960; Joseph, J. (2006), *The Missing Gene: Psychiatry, Heredity, and the Fruitless Search for Genes*, New York: Algora, p. 129; Lewontin et al., 1984. A subsequent 2007 twin study by Prescott et al., found similar results. Prescott et al. (2007), Twin Pair Resemblance for Psychiatric Hospitalization in the Swedish Twin Registry: A 32-Year Follow-Up Study of 29,602 Twin Pairs, *Behavior Genetics, 37*, 547–558. https://doi.org/10.1007/s10519-007-9143-6

20 Joseph, 2004.

21 Kringlen, E. (1976), Twins—Still Our Best Method, *Schizophrenia Bulletin, 2*, 429–433, p. 431. https://doi.org/10.1093/schbul/2.3.429

22 Essen-Möller, E. (1963), Twin Research in Psychiatry, *Acta Psychiatrica Scandinavica, 39*, 65–77, p. 69. https://doi.org/10.1111/j.1600-0447.1963.tb07456.x

23 Shields, J. (1968), Summary of the Genetic Evidence, in D. Rosenthal & S. Kety (Eds.), *The Transmission of Schizophrenia* (pp. 95–126), New York: Pergamon Press, p. 100.

24 Hoffer, A., & Pollin, W. (1970), Schizophrenia in the NAS-NRC Panel of 15,909 Veteran Twin Pairs, *Archives of General Psychiatry, 23*, 469–477. https://doi.org/10.1001/archpsyc.1970.01750050085012, p. 476.

25 Hilker et al. (2017), Heritability of Schizophrenia and Schizophrenia Spectrum Based on the Nationwide Danish Twin Register, *Biological Psychiatry, 83*, 492–498, p. 4, Table 2. https://doi.org/10.1016/j.biopsych.2017.08.017

26 Hilker et al., 2017, p. 6.

27 Hilker et al., 2017, p. 5.

28 Rosenthal, D. (1963), *The Genain Quadruplets: A Study of Heredity and Environment in Schizophrenia*, New York: Basic Books.

29 Rosenthal, 1963. Examples of David Rosenthal's praise for Rüdin and the work of his German psychiatric genetic colleagues are found in Rosenthal, 1970, p. 67; Rosenthal, D. (1971), *Genetics of Psychopathology*, New York: McGraw-Hill, p. 7.

30 DeLisi et al. (1984), The Genain Quadruplets 25 Years Later: A Diagnostic and Biochemical Followup, *Psychiatry Research, 13*, 59–76.

31 Breggin, P. R. (1991), *Toxic Psychiatry*, New York: St. Martins, p. 105.

32 Rosenthal, 1963, p. 9.

33 Rosenthal, 1963, p. 5.

34 I thank Mike Jones for making this point.

35 Hahn, P. D. (2019), *Madness and Genetic Determinism: Is Mental Illness in Our Genes?*, London: Palgrave MacMillan.

36 Rosenthal, 1963, p. 30.

37 Rosenthal, 1963, p. 31.

38 Rosenthal, 1963, p. 34.
39 Rosenthal, 1963, p. 555.
40 Rosenthal, 1963, p. 54.
41 Rosenthal, 1963, p. 56.
42 Rosenthal, 1963, pp. 60–61.
43 Rosenthal, 1963, p. 63.
44 Rosenthal, 1963, p. 69
45 Rosenthal, 1963, p. 78.
46 Rosenthal, 1963, p. 80.
47 Rosenthal, 1963, p. 82.
48 Rosenthal, 1963, p. 84.
49 Rosenthal, 1963, p. 568.
50 Rosenthal, 1963, p. 84.
51 Rosenthal, 1963, p. 87.
52 Rosenthal, 1963, p. 89.
53 Rosenthal, 1963, pp. 90–91.
54 Rosenthal, 1963, pp. 99–100.
55 Rosenthal, 1963, p. 102.
56 Rosenthal, 1963, p. 106.
57 Rosenthal, 1963, p. 108.
58 Rosenthal, 1963, p. 478.
59 Rosenthal, 1963, p. 115.
60 Rosenthal, 1963, p. 116.
61 Rosenthal, 1963, p. 120.
62 Rosenthal, 1963, p. 124.
63 Rosenthal, 1963, p. 125.
64 Rosenthal, 1963, p. 121.
65 Rosenthal, 1963, p. 137.
66 Rosenthal, 1963, p. 121.
67 Rosenthal, 1963, p. 559.
68 Rosenthal, 1963, p. 136.
69 Rosenthal, 1963, p. 146.
70 Rosenthal, 1963, p. 551.
71 Rosenthal, 1963, p. 566.
72 Rosenthal, 1963, p. 559.
73 Rosenthal, 1963, p. 507, 577.
74 Rosenthal, 1963, p. 507, 578.
75 Hahn, 2019, p. 44.
76 van der Kolk, B. A. (2014), *The Body Keeps the Score: Brain, Mind, and Body in the Healing of Trauma*, New York: London: Penguin, p. 30.
77 Gralnick, A. (1942), Folie à Deux—The Psychosis of Association, *Psychiatric Quarterly, 16*, 230–263, p. 232.
78 Jackson, 1960. See also Joseph, J. (2001), Don Jackson's "A Critique of the Literature on the Genetics of Schizophrenia"—A Reappraisal After 40 Years, *Genetic, Social, and General Psychology Monographs, 127*, 27–57. https://pubmed.ncbi.nlm.nih.gov/11352227/
79 Rosenthal, D. (1960), Confusion of Identity and the Frequency of Schizophrenia in Twins, *Archives of General Psychiatry, 3*, 297–304, p. 303. https://doi.org/10.1001/archpsyc.1960.01710030083011
80 Mirsky et al. (2000), A 39-year Follow-up of the Genain Quadruplets, *Schizophrenia Bulletin, 26*, 699–708. https://doi.org/10.1093/oxfordjournals.schbul.a033487
81 DeLisi, L. E. (2017), *100 Questions & Answers about Schizophrenia: Painful Minds* (3rd ed.), Sudbury, MA: Jones & Bartlett, p. 93.

82 Segal, N. L. (2001), Genain Quadruplets: Variations on the Schizophrenic Syndrome, *Twin Research, 4,* 57–59, p. 59. https://doi.org/10.1375/twin.4.1.57
83 Rosenthal, 1963, p. 547.
84 Bentall, R. P. (2009), *Doctoring the Mind: Is Our Current Treatment of Mental Illness Really Any Good?*, New York: New York University Press, p. 117.
85 Mukherjee, S. (2016), *The Gene: An Intimate History*, New York: Scribner.
86 Mukherjee, 2016, p. 387.
87 Joseph, 2004; Teo, T., & Ball, L. C. (2009), Twin Research, Revisionism and Metahistory, *History of the Human Sciences, 22,* 1–23. https://doi.org/10.1177/0952695109345418.
88 Mukherjee, 2016, p. 380.
89 Mukherjee, 2016, pp. 380–381.
90 Mukherjee, 2016, p. 443.
91 Mukherjee, 2016, p. 442. The autism twin study publication cited by Mukherjee was Folstein, S. E., & Rutter, M. (1977), Infantile Autism: A Genetic Study of 21 Twin Pairs, *Journal of Child Psychology and Psychiatry, 18,* 297–321. https://doi.org/10.1111/j.1469-7610.1977.tb00443.x
92 Mukherjee, 2016, p. 298.
93 Mukherjee, 2016, p. 298.
94 Mukherjee, 2016, p. 298.
95 The original NAS schizophrenia twin study was Pollin et al. (1969), Psychopathology in 15,909 Pairs of Veteran Twins: Evidence for a Genetic Factor in the Pathogenesis of Schizophrenia and its Relative Absence in Psychoneurosis, *American Journal of Psychiatry, 126,* 597–610. https://doi.org/10.1176/ajp.126.5.597
96 Kendler, K. S., & Robinette, C. D. (1983), Schizophrenia in the National Academy of Sciences-National Research Council Twin Registry: A 16-year Update, *American Journal of Psychiatry, 140,* 1551–1563. https://doi.org/10.1176/ajp.140.12.1551
97 Pollin et al., 1969, p. 608.
98 Hilker et al., 2017, p. 1.
99 Mukherjee, 2016, p. 443.
100 Mukherjee, 2016, pp. 442–443.
101 Koskenvuo et al. (1984), Psychiatric Hospitalization in Twins, *Acta Geneticae Medicae et Gemellologiae, 33,* 321–332, p. 321. https://doi.org/10.1017/S0001566000007364
102 Sullivan et al., 2003, p. 1188.
103 Joseph, J. (2016, June 2), Reared-Apart Twin Study Mythology: The Latest Contribution (Part One), Web log post, *Mad in America,* https://www.madinamerica.com/2016/06/reared-apart-twin-study-mythology-the-latest-contri-bution-part-1/; Joseph, J. (2016, June 27), Reared-Apart Twin Study Mythology: The Latest Contribution (Part Two), https://www.madinamerica.com/2016/06/reared-apart-twin-study-mythology-the-latest-contribution-part-two/.
104 Joseph, 2016 Part One, Part Two.
105 In "Ken Burns Presents *The Gene: An Intimate History,*" the schizophrenia segment is found in Part II, 50:50–53:02.
106 Mukherjee, 2016, p. 443.
107 Fischer, M. (1971), Psychoses in the Offspring of Schizophrenic Monozygotic Twins and their Normal Co-Twins, *British Journal of Psychiatry, 118,* 43–51. https://doi.org/10.1192/bjp.118.542.43; Gottesman, I. I., & Bertelsen, A. (1989), Confirming Unexpressed Genotypes for Schizophrenia, *Archives of General Psychiatry, 46,* 867–872. https://doi.org/10.1001/archpsyc.1989.01810100009002

108 Kringlen, E., & Cramer, G. (1989), Offspring of Monozygotic Twins Discordant for Schizophrenia, *Archives of General Psychiatry, 46,* 873–877. https://doi.org /10.1001/archpsyc.1989.01810100015003

109 Torrey, E. F. (1990), Offspring of Twins with Schizophrenia [Letter to the Editor], *Archives of General Psychiatry, 47,* 976–977. https://doi.org/10.1001/ archpsyc.1990.01810220092013

110 For a critical analysis of research on the offspring of discordant MZ pairs, see Joseph, 1998, *A Critical Analysis of the Genetic Theory of Schizophrenia*; Joseph, 2004, pp. 187–193.

111 Farber, S. L. (1981), *Identical Twins Reared Apart: A Reanalysis,* New York: Basic Books, Chapter 6.

112 Craike, W. H., & Slater, E. (1945), Folie à Deux in Uniovular Twins Reared Apart, *Brain, 68, Part III*, 213–221.

113 Craike & Slater, 1945, pp. 219, 221.

114 Taylor, H. F. (1980), *The IQ Game: A Methodological Inquiry into the Heredity-Environment Controversy*, New Brunswick, NJ: Rutgers University Press. See also Joseph, 2015.

115 Gottesman, I. I. (1982), [Review of the Book *Identical Twins Reared Apart: A Reanalysis*, by S. Farber], *American Journal of Psychology, 95,* 350–352, p. 351.

116 Kendler, K. S. (1993), Twin Studies of Psychiatric Illness: Current Status and Future Directions, *Archives of General Psychiatry, 50,* 905–915, p. 907. https:// doi.org/10.1001/archpsyc.1993.01820230075007

117 Kenneth Kendler's first major defense of the EEA and psychiatric twin studies was published in 1983. Kendler, K. S. (1983), Overview: A Current Perspective on Twin Studies of Schizophrenia, *American Journal of Psychiatry, 140,* 1413–1425. https://doi.org/10.1176/ajp.140.11.1413

6 Schizophrenia Adoption Research

I now turn to the important area of schizophrenia adoption research. Contemporary readers might wonder why I will spend so many pages examining studies published decades ago. There are two main reasons. The first is that in the 1960s and 1970s, these adoption studies played a major role in supporting genetic theories of schizophrenia and psychosis, theories that we have seen remain dominant to this day, and in the process were seen as legitimizing and validating the earlier twin studies. But just as important, the most frequently cited schizophrenia adoption studies provide case histories of how massively flawed research, where investigators dismissed or minimized the impact of environmental confounds, openly manipulated data to match confirmation biases, and changed definitions and comparison groups as they went along to reach desired conclusions, remain pillars of psychiatric theories and claims. Such practices may have been acceptable at the time, but they are not acceptable now.

A wise person once said, "Data don't tell stories, scientists tell stories."[1] In the replication crisis era, previously accepted stories researchers told about their data are receiving increasing attention and scrutiny. The language developed since the early 2010s to describe unsound research practices has enabled those of us with perspectives that differ from mainstream behavioral science positions to tell *our* stories in new and better ways. In the previous chapters my analysis was more about problems with research methods than with specific studies. The schizophrenia adoption research critique requires a greater emphasis on deconstructing the individual studies. By necessity I will describe how these studies were performed in some detail, and I will approach them from the questionable research practices (QRP) perspective, which was not in existence when my previous analyses were published.[2] It is not a deconstruction story that psychiatry and psychiatric genetics want to hear—since it argues for overturning everything these fields have said about schizophrenia adoption research for the past half-century— but it is a story that must be told.

Psychiatric adoption studies are based on the idea that genetic and environmental influences on behavior are completely separated (disentangled)

DOI: 10.4324/9781003293279-6

by the adoption process, and that the adoption process itself does not psychologically affect or harm children in ways that could bias a study's results. Before looking at the individual studies, I will address these issues.

Separation of Genes and Environment?

Abandoned Children

Because family and twin studies have been rightfully criticized since their inception as being unable to separate the potential influences of genes and environment, schizophrenia adoption studies were developed with the aim of finally achieving this separation. Researchers performing these studies believed that the adoption process accomplishes this separation because adoptees inherit the genes of their biological (birth) parents, but are reared in the environment of another (adoptive) family with whom they share no genetic relationship. From the perspective of schizophrenia adoption researcher David Rosenthal, who we remember from Chapter 5 as the lead investigator/author of the Genain Quadruplets study, adoption studies "separate the genetic and rearing variables entirely."[3] But is this really the case?

"Adoptees" in schizophrenia adoption research were children abandoned by, or taken from, their birthparent(s) for various reasons, often under difficult conditions in early-to-mid 20th-century Europe and the United States. It is likely that most experienced attachment-rupture trauma, emotional suffering, loneliness and neglect, abuse, poverty, and other adverse childhood conditions. This was especially true for the late-separated children, and for children who spent time in an orphanage. Adoption placements are not made randomly, and these studies were subject to the "selective placement" biases I will discuss after describing the individual studies.

A more fitting name for this area of research is the *study of abandoned children*, a term that places emphasis on the conditions children experience between birth and their eventual placement with an adoptive family, and the psychological impact these experiences may have had throughout a person's life.[4] Research performed since the 1990s has shown that disturbed or ruptured parent-child attachment patterns can influence brain development during critical developmental periods.[5] These findings call into question adoption researchers' claim that their conclusions apply (generalize) to the population of non-adoptees.

In addition to sharing a prenatal environment with their often-stressed birthmother, during sensitive developmental periods, most people studied in schizophrenia adoption research, as children, (1) were reared for a certain period by their biological parent(s); (2) suffered a disruption of attachment bonds with their biological parent(s); and/or (3) may have been placed into unstable or psychologically/developmentally harmful environments, such as foster homes and orphanages, between separation and adoption.

Even children adopted away at birth share several environmental factors in common with their birthmothers. These always include the prenatal environment (including prenatal nutrition and the mother's possible chemical dependency), usually include skin color and "race" (frequently leading to oppression or privilege), and often include similar physical appearance, social class, culture, religion, and so on. For these reasons alone, Rosenthal was mistaken when he said that adoption studies "separate the genetic and rearing variables entirely."

Range Restriction and Representativeness

Couples that adopt children are not representative of the full range of family homes in the population. Kenneth Kendler and his psychiatric genetic colleague Pak Sham discussed "several potential methodological limitations" in psychiatric adoption research, one of which is "unrepresentativeness." This refers to the fact that "biological parents who give children up for adoption ... have higher rates of psychiatric illness and drug problems (although several generations ago, a more likely problem was poverty)." In contrast, "adoptive parents are typically mentally healthier than the general populace because adoption agencies see it as their job to select 'healthy' families in which to place their adoptees."[6] Because agencies usually screen potential adoptive parents for mental health problems, it is not surprising that adoption studies find fewer psychiatric disorders among them.

I will now describe the original schizophrenia adoption studies, followed by a discussion of how the adoption process in each of the countries where these studies were performed was influenced by the social conditions in which adoptions were made. I will then perform a critical analysis of the two most frequently cited studies, followed by a discussion of problems in textbooks and other secondary source descriptions of these studies.

The Schizophrenia Adoption Studies

Leonard Heston's U.S. Oregon Study

In 1966, genetically oriented psychiatric researcher Leonard Heston assessed the rate of schizophrenia among the 47 adopted-away biological offspring of women diagnosed with schizophrenia, who were confined to Oregon (United States) state mental hospitals.[7] Heston, who was not blind to the group status of the adoptees, along with 2 colleagues, made 5 schizophrenia diagnoses among these 47 experimental group adoptees, versus 0 among the 50 control adoptees, a result that reached statistical significance ($p = .024$).

Heston concluded that his results "strongly support a genetic aetiology of schizophrenia."[8]

This study was subject to the general problems of psychiatric adoption research, in addition to the questionable research practices I discussed in Chapter 1. Like all research of that era, Heston was able to make decisions behind the scenes and present a paper for publication with little accountability related to how he made decisions. The study appeared in the *British Journal of Psychiatry*, then edited by Munich-trained psychiatric geneticist Eliot Slater. Like Slater, Heston supported the single-gene theory of causation.[9] The reported *p*-value for the experimental versus control group comparison was one diagnosis away from being statistically non-significant.[10]

Other selected problems specific to Heston's study include the following points: (1) schizophrenia was not defined. Heston stated only that schizophrenia diagnoses were made "conservatively," and were based on "generally accepted standards."[11] (2) No attempt was made to assess the psychiatric status of the biological fathers. (3) Only one brief case history was provided, which made independent analysis of adoptees' history and mental/diagnostic status difficult. (4) About 25 percent of the adoptees were not interviewed, yet were retained in the study. (5) Almost half of the adoptees had spent months or years in an orphanage, with Heston admitting that "none of the subjects [was] reared in typical or 'normal' circumstances."[12] (6) As I will soon discuss, the results were biased by selective placement factors. I have reviewed problems with Heston's study in more detail elsewhere.[13]

The Danish-American Studies

The Danish-American adoption studies were performed in the 1960s–1990s by American psychiatric researchers Seymour Kety, David Rosenthal, Paul Wender, and their Danish colleagues who included Fini Schulsinger and Joseph Welner. These are the most frequently cited schizophrenia adoption studies, and are therefore the main focus of this chapter. Seymour Kety (1915–2000) was a highly regarded psychiatric researcher who had developed the first quantitative technique for measuring blood flow in the living brain. Kety first proposed the idea of performing an adoption study of schizophrenia in a 1959 article published in *Science*.[14] In 1999, Kety won a "Special Achievement in Medical Science" Lasker Award. (The Lasker is sometimes referred to as the "American Nobel.") We have seen that David Rosenthal (who passed away in 1996) was a psychologist at the U.S. National Institute of Mental Health. Paul Wender (1934–2016) was a psychiatrist who later was involved in ADHD research. In 1962, Kety, Rosenthal, and Wender decided to pool their efforts, and with Schulsinger's help they began the study in Denmark in 1963.[15]

The investigators used three different research designs. Using the *Adoptees' Family Study* design, the Kety-led studies began with adoptees as first-identified relatives (see Figure 6.1). We have seen that in the psychiatric genetics literature, the first-identified relatives are often referred to as "probands." Using the *Adoptees Study* design, like Heston, the Rosenthal-led study began with biological parents as the first-identified relatives or probands (see Figure 6.2). Using the third *Crossfostering Study* design, Wender and colleagues studied the adopted-away biological offspring of Danish parents not diagnosed with schizophrenia, but who were raised by an adoptive parent eventually diagnosed with a schizophrenia spectrum disorder.[16] Diagnoses in this group were then compared with other groups. Because the Kety-led and Rosenthal-led studies are the most frequently cited Danish-American studies, in this chapter I will focus on these two studies and refer readers to critics' analyses of the very problematic Crossfostering Study.[17]

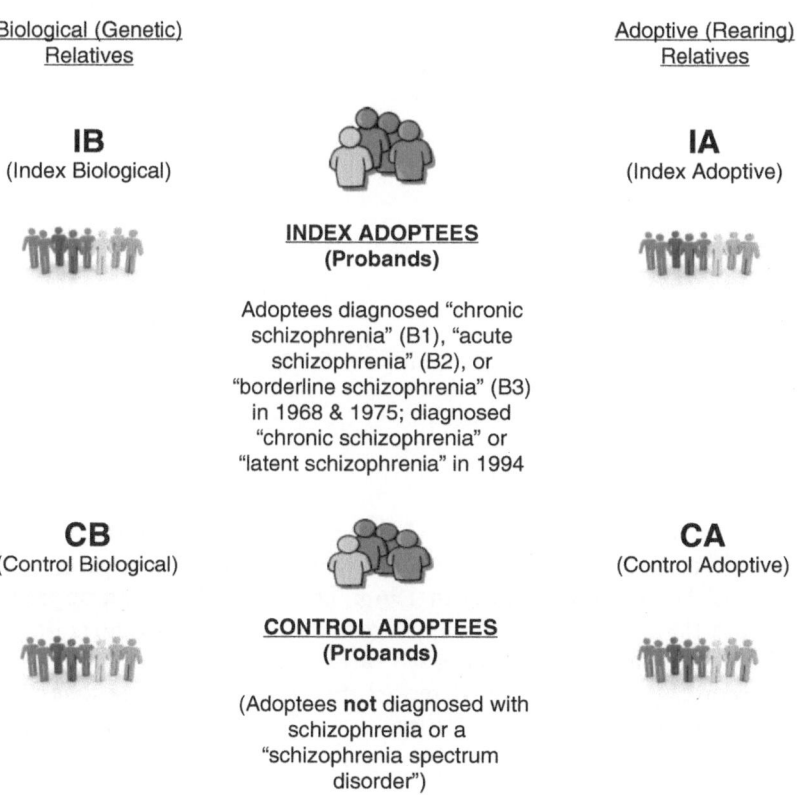

Figure 6.1 The Kety-led "Adoptees' Family Study" Probands and Relatives

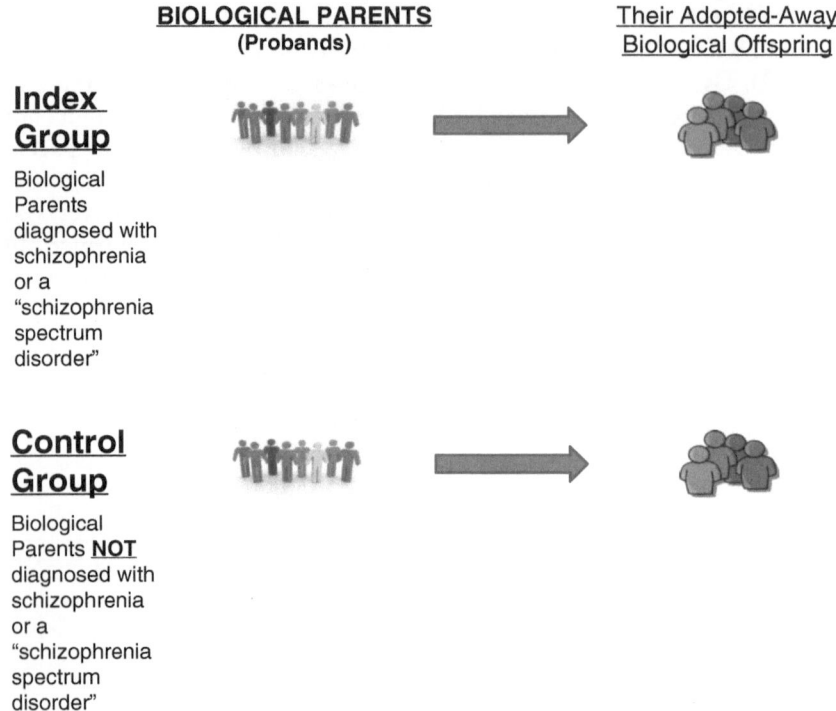

Results based on comparing schizophrenia spectrum diagnoses
in the index versus control biological-offspring groups

BIOLOGICAL PARENTS
(Probands)

Their Adopted-Away
Biological Offspring

**Index
Group**

Biological
Parents
diagnosed with
schizophrenia
or a
"schizophrenia
spectrum
disorder"

**Control
Group**

Biological
Parents **NOT**
diagnosed with
schizophrenia
or a
"schizophrenia
spectrum
disorder"

Figure 6.2 The Rosenthal-led Study's "Adoptees Study" Design (also used in the
Heston and Tienari-led studies)

The Kety-led Study

The most frequently cited Danish-American adoption study is Kety,
Rosenthal, Wender, and colleagues' study carried out in two geographical regions of Denmark beginning in 1963. The first publication appeared
in 1968, and the final publication appeared in 1994. In both parts of this
study, the preliminary report was based on diagnoses obtained from institutional records, while in the final report the researchers made diagnoses
based on interviewing available relatives.

The 1968 Records-based Copenhagen Study

The original 1968 "Copenhagen Study" began with the records of 5,483
Danish children adopted by non-relatives in the city and county of
Copenhagen between 1924 and 1947.[18] Of these adopted children, records

from Danish psychiatric registers identified 507 who later in life had been admitted to a Danish psychiatric facility for any reason. Based on these records, the researchers diagnosed 33 adoptees with "chronic," "acute," or "borderline (latent)" schizophrenia.[19] These became the 33 "index adoptee" probands. The researchers also established a control group, which consisted of 33 adoptees with no record of admission to a Danish psychiatric facility. Each control adoptee was matched to an index adoptee based on age, sex, socioeconomic status of the rearing family, and other factors. Kety and colleagues then made blind, consensus diagnoses among the 306 identified first- and second-degree biological relatives of these index and control adoptees (150 index, 156 control). They performed the same procedure for the 157 index and control adoptive (rearing) relatives. The four groups of relatives are seen in Figure 6.1. Based on finding a statistically significant schizophrenia spectrum disorder rate in the index biological relative group compared with the control biological relative group, Kety and colleagues concluded that "genetic factors are important in the transmission of schizophrenia."[20]

The 1975 Interview-based Copenhagen Study

In a widely cited 1975 follow-up study, the researchers assessed the diagnostic status of the 1968 Copenhagen biological and adoptive relatives, but here they did so using psychiatric interviews.[21] These were the first- and second-degree relatives of the 33 index and 33 control adoptees identified in the 1968 study, although the control group now consisted of 34 adoptees.[22] The biological relative group had now grown to 347 (173 index, 174 control). The researchers undertook the difficult task of tracking down and attempting to interview these relatives. They believed there were many more "schizophrenia-related disorders" among them that had not come to the attention of mental health facilities or hospitals, and were therefore unrecorded in the 1968 study. The interviews were conducted by the Danish members of the research team, and were written up in English as 35-page transcripts. These transcripts were edited to remove information that could reveal the relative's group status, and were sent to Kety, Wender, and Rosenthal in the United States, who made blind "consensus" psychiatric diagnoses. The code was then broken and the relatives (and their possible diagnoses) were allocated to their respective groups as defined by their relationship to the index and control adoptees. Based on finding a significantly higher number of schizophrenia spectrum disorders among the index biological versus the control biological relative groups, in addition to other comparisons, the researchers concluded that their results were "strongly suggestive of the operation of genetic factors."[23]

The Provincial Study

After the completion of the Copenhagen 1968 records-based and 1975 interview-based studies, the researchers extended their investigation to the remaining provinces of Denmark. The preliminary records-based results of this "Provincial Study" were published in 1978. The final interview-based Provincial Study results were not published until 1994.[24] In their 1994 publication, the researchers combined the Copenhagen and Provincial results to produce the "Danish National Sample." Kety and colleagues concluded in 1994 that their findings "provide important and necessary support for the assumption often made in family studies: observed familial clustering in schizophrenia is an expression of shared genetic factors."[25]

The Rosenthal-led Study

Unlike the Kety-led studies, which began with adoptees as the first-identified relative (proband), in the Rosenthal-led study the first-identified relatives were parents who had given up a child for adoption. The first publication appeared in 1968, which was followed by a 1971 publication based on an enlarged sample.[26] The researchers began with the records of the same 5,483 Danish adoptees identified in the Kety-led study, and then identified around 10,000 of their biological parents.

As stated in their original 1968 publication, the purpose of the study was to identify components of the "assumed diathesis" (predisposition) of schizophrenia. Rosenthal et al., assumed in advance that "heredity was an important contributor to schizophrenia." Another stated assumption of the study was that "this inherited factor manifested itself in the behavior or personality of persons who were not frankly schizophrenic."[27]

Based on institutional records, Rosenthal and colleagues identified 76 Danish biological parents (50 mothers, 26 fathers) who they diagnosed with "schizophrenia," "doubtful schizophrenia," or "manic-depressive psychosis."[28] The 76 adopted-away biological offspring of these parents constituted the index adoptee group. The researchers compared the diagnostic rate found in this adopted-away offspring group to a matched control group consisting of the 67 adopted-away offspring of parents with no known psychiatric history. The Rosenthal-led study's basic design, also used in the Heston- and Tienari-led studies, is seen in Figure 6.2.

In lieu of a consensus diagnosis of each adoptee, in the 1968 and 1971 studies the researchers used what they called "thumbnail diagnostic formulations."[29] All 1968 and 1971 diagnoses, statistical comparisons, and conclusions in favor of genetics were based on these formulations, which were prepared by Welner and Schulsinger based on a 3–5-hour interview with each adoptee. Examples of thumbnail diagnostic formulations that counted as schizophrenia in the 1971 study included "possible paranoid borderline," "paranoid character," "almost pseudoneurotic borderline," "moderately schizoid," "pronounced preschizophrenic diathesis," and "conceivably paranoid borderline."[30] In their 1971 publication, Rosenthal and colleagues calculated a 31.6 percent (24/76) rate "in the schizophrenia spectrum" thumbnail diagnostics among the index adoptees, versus a 17.8 percent (12/67) rate among the control adoptees.[31] This comparison reached statistical significance just below the .05 level, allowing them to conclude, "The authors believe that evidence from this study supports the theory that heredity plays a significant role in the etiology of schizophrenia spectrum disorders."[32] As I will discuss later, Rosenthal and colleagues presented their consensus schizophrenia spectrum diagnoses for the first and final time in a 1978 publication.[33]

The Tienari-led Finnish Study

In contrast to the Heston and Danish-American investigations, Pekka Tienari (1931–2018) and colleagues' 1980s–2000s "Finnish Adoptive Family Study of Schizophrenia" took the important step of looking at adoptive family environments as well as adoptees' genetic background.[34] Like the Heston and Rosenthal-led studies, Tienari and colleagues began with diagnosed parents as the first-identified relatives. Their index group consisted of the 190 adopted-away biological offspring of mothers diagnosed with DSM-III-R schizophrenia and other "schizophrenia spectrum disorders." Tienari and colleagues reported a statistically significant index versus control difference for the "schizophrenia spectrum" disorders combined. For "typical schizophrenia" alone, however, there was no statistically significant index versus control group difference.[35] They concluded that in addition to genetic background, adoptive family environments "were a significant predictor of schizophrenia spectrum disorders in adoptees."[36]

In addition to the general problems of psychiatric adoption research, and the questionable research practices of that era, selected problems specific to Tienari's study include (1) the above-mentioned failure to find a statistically significant index versus control schizophrenia difference, (2) about one-third of the adoptees were placed after their mother was diagnosed with a psychotic disorder,[37] (3) the definition of schizophrenia was broadened to include "schizophrenia spectrum disorders," (4) some adoptees were placed in their adoptive family as late as age four,[38] and (5) the results were biased by selective placement factors (see below).[39] Detailed critical analyses of the Tienari-led study are available elsewhere.[40]

The Lichtenstein-led Swedish Study

In 2009, Paul Lichtenstein and colleagues performed a large study of relative risks in Sweden, based on records obtained from a population register and a hospital discharge register. Their main purpose was to assess whether schizophrenia and bipolar disorder "share common genetic determinants." When studying adoptive relationships, they found an elevated schizophrenia risk among the adopted-away biological offspring of parents diagnosed with schizophrenia as well as among the adopted-away siblings of non-adopted siblings. Lichtenstein and colleagues did not use an adoption control group.

They did not state how many adoptees they studied, or provide information relating to adoptees' placement or age at separation.[41] In addition to parent/adopted-away offspring pairs, the Lichtenstein-led study calculated sibling/adopted-away sibling risks.

Selective Placement Bias

A major additional factor casting doubt on the idea that psychiatric adoption studies can separate the potential influences of genes and environments is these studies' often-unstated "no selective placement assumption." Because children are not randomly assigned to available adoptive homes and then observed as they are growing up, researchers must *assume* that factors relating to the adoption process (including the policies of adoption agencies) did not lead to the systematic placement of certain types of children into environments contributing to a higher rate of the disorder in question.

Most adoptees were placed in the early-to-middle part of the 20th century in Denmark, the United States (Oregon), and Finland. The Swedish study index relatives and adoptees were born between 1932 and 2002. Although rarely mentioned by the original investigators or by the authors of secondary sources, all four regions had laws permitting the forced eugenic sterilization of people labeled "schizophrenic," "insane," "feeble-minded," and so on. Large segments of society in that era, including adoption agencies, followed the lead of authorities such as Kraepelin, Bleuler, Rüdin, Luxenburger, Kallmann and many others who believed that the offspring of people with schizophrenia or "insanity" in their family background were the undesirable carriers of "hereditary taint."

Denmark

In 1929 Denmark became the first European nation to pass a eugenics-inspired sterilization law.[42] This law (a stronger law was passed in 1935) was in force until well after the last studied Danish adoptees were placed. Placements in the Danish-American studies were made between 1924 and 1947, an era that included the Great Depression and World War II. The forced sterilization of the "insane" and other "eugenically undesirable" people in Denmark continued into the 1960s.[43]

The Danish adoption agencies checked a potential adoptee's genetic family background to determine his or her suitability (or desirability) for adoption. As seen in the 1946–1947 annual report of the Mother's Aid Organization of Copenhagen, which was the largest adoption service in the country, the Danish authorities believed that a future adoptee's genetic "developmental potential" was "of great importance" for the "correct placement" of the child.[44]

When Danish agencies suspected a family history of mental disorders, they consulted the Danish Institute of Human Genetics, which was the keeper of the Danish National Psychiatric Register. The Register was established in 1937, and included the names of people diagnosed with mental disorders, and people who had been psychiatrically hospitalized.[45] It was created at a time when support for eugenic ideas and practices were at their high point in Denmark (and in the world as a whole). The Psychiatric Register, which enabled the Danish-American adoption studies to be performed, was created to aid eugenic programs and eugenics-influenced adoption placement decisions.[46]

According to genetic researcher Sarnoff Mednick, "Every weekend (at least in the 1930s), Danish people who wished to adopt would visit the orphanages and pick children.... Children whose selection by an adoptive parent is delayed may be less attractive physically and behaviorally."[47] Many children were also perceived as being less attractive *genetically*. Clearly, the most loving and emotionally stable potential adoptive parents, who were usually informed of "deviance" in the adoptee's biological family background, would not have picked children "tainted" by a family history of mental disorders.

Oregon (USA)

Similar conditions existed in Oregon, where Heston's adoptees were placed between 1915 and 1945. Although Heston did not mention this in his adoption study publications, Oregon passed a law in 1917 creating a "State Board of Eugenics," whose duty was to authorize the compulsory sterilization of "all feeble-minded, insane, epileptic, habitual criminals, moral degenerates and sexual perverts," because they might produce "inferior" offspring.[48] An additional 1919 Oregon law stipulated that if a person had been admitted to a mental hospital, this constituted "prima facie evidence that procreation by any such person would produce children with an inherited tendency to feeble-mindedness, insanity, epilepsy, criminality or degeneracy."[49] The author of a 1925 article in *Eugenical News* wrote approvingly that, whereas sterilization laws in many U.S. states were limited to "inmates of institutions," in Oregon "there is a Eugenics Commissioner, who has authority to comb the state for degenerates and enforce sterilization."[50] Because Heston's index adoptees were born to women hospitalized with schizophrenia, it is very unlikely that the "tainted" children they gave birth to were placed into the same types of adoptive homes as were the "non-tainted" control children.

Finland and Sweden

In 1935 the Finnish Parliament passed the Sterilization Act, which allowed the compulsory eugenic sterilization and castration of "idiots," "imbeciles," and the "insane," which included people carrying the schizophrenia and manic-depression labels.[51] In 1950, Finland passed the Castration

Act, which permitted the castration of criminals, the mentally retarded, and the "permanently mentally ill." Compulsory eugenic sterilization was not legally abolished in Finland until 1970. Sweden also had a long history of eugenics and compulsory eugenic sterilization.[52]

***

The evidence strongly suggests that schizophrenia adoption studies' critical "no selective placement assumption" was violated in all studies published to date. Children with a biological family history of mental disorders were seen as inferior potential adoptees, and it is therefore likely that they were placed into more chaotic, exploitative, and psychologically harmful (and potentially more "schizophrenogenic") adoptive families. Once again, potential environmental and genetic influences in psychiatric genetic research are difficult to disentangle.

Having touched on problems relating to the design and logic of psychiatric adoption studies, I will now describe major problem areas in the two most frequently cited schizophrenia adoption studies in the context of the QRP concept described in Chapter 1.

Major Problem Areas in the Danish-American Adoption Studies

We saw in Chapter 1 that in 2015 the "Open Science Collaboration" team found that only 36 percent of the surveyed psychological studies could be independently replicated at a statistically significant level.[53] Some explanations for this finding, according to the investigators, included QRPs that I will show were common in the Danish-American adoption studies: "Selective reporting, selective analysis, and insufficient specification of the conditions necessary or sufficient to obtain the results."[54]

The Danish-American Kety-led and Rosenthal-led studies have been the subject of several major critical reviews.[55] They were also the focus of several "independent" analyses, performed by genetically oriented psychiatrists and psychologists in the 1980s and 1990s, who re-analyzed the original Danish-American adoption study data based on supposedly superior 1980 DSM-III "operationalized" diagnostic criteria.[56] These analyses, which were published in leading psychiatry journals, are often cited in textbooks as having "reaffirmed" or "upheld" the original Danish-American findings. I will not focus on these analyses in this chapter because I will argue that the original studies themselves produced no genetic findings to reaffirm.

The 1968 Danish-American Diagnostic Process

Unlike the 1980 DSM-III through the 2022 DSM-5TR (Fifth Edition, Text Revision) diagnostic criteria, which were based on the more objective (yet still problematic[57]) method of checking off a list of symptoms, the

Danish-American researchers diagnosed adoptees and relatives using the older "global" (or "consensus") diagnostic system based on 1968 DSM-II descriptions.[58] They described the method they used to arrive at a diagnosis, which they used in the entire series spanning more than 25 years, as follows:

> Four copies of the edited summary were prepared and distributed to the four authors who served as raters and who independently characterized each subject according to the classification described below [see Table 6.2]. The individual ratings were then tabulated and those cases in which there was disagreement among the raters were discussed at a conference of all four authors where an effort was made to review additional edited information which it was possible to obtain and to arrive at a consensus diagnosis acceptable to all. In 4 cases there remained an evenly split opinion regarding the presence of schizophrenia or doubtful schizophrenia, and these were not included in those categories.[59]

Although Kety claimed "a high degree" of diagnostic reliability in his studies, each investigator approached the diagnostic process somewhat differently.[60] According to Kety, each rater's "individual definitions of schizophrenia varied by virtue of [their] training and experience, from a substantial reliance on Kraepelin and Bleuler to the broader psychodynamic concepts which were taught in the 50s."[61]

Psychiatric diagnoses in that era were described by Flint, Greenspan, and Kendler in 2020 as "not that reliable...Diagnostic manuals contained vague descriptions of psychiatric disorders, open to varying interpretations."[62] In a 2022 schizophrenia research review article appearing in *The Lancet*, Sameer Jauhar and colleagues wrote that after World War II, "the concept of schizophrenia was broadened to the point of near meaninglessness."[63] As I will show, the Danish-American researchers turned the production of unreliable, vague, non-psychotic, and near-meaningless definitions of schizophrenia into an artform.

The Schizophrenia Spectrum Concept

We have seen that the Danish-American investigators decided to expand the definition of schizophrenia to include what they called *schizophrenia spectrum disorders*. As described in the 1968 Kety-led study, the Danish-American schizophrenia spectrum consisted of "chronic schizophrenia" (which the researchers called "B1"), "acute schizophrenia reaction" ("B2"), "borderline schizophrenia" ("B3"; also called "latent schizophrenia"), "uncertain chronic schizophrenia" ("D1"), "uncertain acute schizophrenia reaction" ("D2"), "uncertain borderline schizophrenia" ("D3"), and "inadequate personality" ("C"; called "schizoid or inadequate personality" in the 1975 study). The researchers decided to count all these, including the "inadequate personality" and "uncertain" relatives, as schizophrenia. The 1968 Danish-American schizophrenia spectrum is seen in Table 6.1.

The 1968 Kety-led study index group consisted of 16 B1, 7 B2, and 10 B3 adoptees, for a total of 33. The 1975 study was based on the same index and control adoptees, but one index B3 diagnosis was changed to B1 based on an interview. The 1975 index group therefore consisted of 17 B1, 7 B2, and 9 B3 adoptees. The researchers grouped together the B diagnoses (B1, B2, and B3) and called them "definite schizophrenia." They grouped together the D diagnoses (D1, D2, and D3) and called them "uncertain schizophrenia." Table 6.2 contains Kety and colleagues' complete description of their Copenhagen spectrum categories, as seen in their original 1968 publication.

We see in Table 6.2 that the "B" diagnostic categories captured vaguely defined behaviors, with the "D" diagnoses representing "uncertain" versions of these categories. In Kety and colleagues' own words, "uncertain schizophrenia" was a "vague and subjective category, which hardly qualifies as schizophrenia according to our own or other criteria."[65] Elsewhere they recognized that their spectrum diagnoses were "necessarily vague,"[66] with a "lack of sharp boundaries."[67] The global diagnostic system did not require adoptees or relatives to display a standard number of these behaviors, or even the same behaviors.

In the Kety-led 1968 and 1975 studies, the researchers selected as index adoptees (probands) only those with B "definite schizophrenia" conditions (see the bolded diagnoses in Table 6.1). Diagnoses among the *relatives*, on the other hand, included the B, D "uncertain schizophrenia," and C "inadequate personality/schizoid" conditions. The researchers' decision to expand the definition of schizophrenia in the four relative groups enabled them to find more spectrum diagnoses among these relatives. In their original 1968 and 1975 publications, Kety and colleagues said that the issue was about fine-tuning the schizophrenia spectrum in the relative groups, when in fact

Table 6.1 1968 Danish-American Schizophrenia
                Spectrum Diagnoses Made on Relatives

---

*Diagnoses Counted as Schizophrenia in the
1968 Kety-led Study*

B1. Chronic Schizophrenia
B2. Acute Schizophrenia Reaction
B3. Borderline Schizophrenia
D1. Uncertain Chronic Schizophrenia
D2. Uncertain Acute Schizophrenia Reaction
D3. Uncertain Borderline Schizophrenia
C. Inadequate Personality

All diagnoses given to relatives. Adoptee probands (bold type) diagnosed B1, B2, and B3 only.

Table 6.2 The 1968 Danish-American Schizophrenia Spectrum as Described by Kety, Rosenthal, Wender, and Colleagues[64]

B1.	"Chronic Schizophrenia ('chronic undifferentiated schizophrenia,' 'true schizophrenia,' 'process schizophrenia'). *Characteristics:* (1) Poor pre-psychotic adjustment; introverted; schizoid; shut-in; few peer contacts; few heterosexual contacts; usually unmarried; poor occupational adjustment. (2) Onset—gradual and without clear-cut psychological precipitant. (3) Presenting picture: presence of primary Bleulerian characteristics; presence of clear rather than confused sensorium. (4) Post- hospital course—failure to reach previous level of adjustment. (5) Tendency to chronicity."
B2.	"Acute schizophrenic reaction (acute undifferentiated schizophrenic reaction, schizo- affective psychosis, possible schizophreniform psychosis, (acute) paranoid reaction, homosexual panic). *Characteristics:* (1) Relatively good premorbid adjustment. (2) Relatively rapid onset of illness with clear-cut psychological precipitant. (3) Presenting picture: presence of secondary symptoms and comparatively lesser evidence of primary ones; presence of affect (manic-depressive symptoms, feelings of guilt); cloudy rather than clear sensorium. (4) Post-hospital course good. (5) Tendency to relatively brief episode(s) responding to drugs, EST, etc."
B3.	"Border-line state (pseudoneurotic schizophrenia, border-line, ambulatory schizophrenia, questionable simple schizophrenia, 'psychotic character,' severe schizoid individual). *Characteristics:* (1) Thinking: strange or atypical mentation; thought shows tendency to ignore reality, logic and experience (to an excessive degree) resulting in poor adaptation to life experience (despite the presence of normal IQ); fuzzy, murky, vague speech. (2) Experience: brief episodes of cognitive distortion (the patient can, and does, snap back but during the episode the idea has more the character of a delusion than an ego-alien obsessive thought); feelings of depersonalization, of strangeness or unfamiliarity with or toward the familiar; micropsychosis, (3) Affective: anhedonia—never experiences intense pleasure—never happy; no deep or intense involvement with anyone or anybody. (4) Interpersonal behavior: may appear poised, but lacking depth ('as if' personality); sexual adjustment: chaotic fluctuation, mixture of hetero- and homosexuality. (5) Psychopathology: multiple neurotic manifestations which shift frequently (obsessive concerns, phobias, conversion, psychosomatic symptoms, etc.); severe widespread anxiety."
C.	"Inadequate personality. *Characteristics:* A somewhat heterogeneous group consisting of individuals who would be classified as either inadequate of schizoid by the *APA Diagnostic Manual* [DSM-II]. Persons so classified often had many of the characteristics of the B3 category, but to a considerably milder degree."
D1, 2 or 3	"Uncertain B1, 2, or 3 either because information is lacking or because even if enough information is available, the case does not fit clearly into an appropriate B category."

it was about *expanding* it. "Schizophrenia," therefore, was defined in very different ways within the same study, depending on whether the researchers were diagnosing proband adoptees or their relatives.

Necessity of Broadening the Definition of Schizophrenia

The researchers decided to broaden the definition of schizophrenia to include schizophrenia spectrum disorders (1) to have enough cases to be able to conduct their studies and (2) to create the possibility of finding a statistically significant index schizophrenia elevation versus the control group after no such elevation was found using only the original B1 "chronic" definition of schizophrenia. As Rosenthal acknowledged, he and his colleagues "broaden[ed] the concept of schizophrenic disorder as widely as it may have ever been reasonably conceived before."[68] An example of just how far Rosenthal was willing to broaden the definition of schizophrenia is seen in this 1979 statement:

> For every hospitalizable schizophrenic, there are many more people in the community who have a schizophrenic-like type of disorder which is not severe enough to require hospitalization. These individuals are called borderline or pseudoneurotic schizophrenic, schizoid, paranoid, or simply cold, distant and inadequate, or odd and eccentric.[69]

The investigators created the spectrum after finding, in the 1968 Kety-led study, only 16 adoptee probands with B1 chronic schizophrenia among the 5,483 identified adoptees (about 0.3%), when 38–40 adoptee B1 diagnoses would have been expected based on a Danish age-corrected lifetime risk of 0.7 percent.[70] This sample of 16 B1 chronic schizophrenia adoptees was, as Rosenthal acknowledged, a "lower than expected yield,"[71] which was "too small to make any of these studies meaningful."[72]

This "lower than expected yield" adoptee proband B1 schizophrenia rate showed that being reared by adoptive parents screened by Danish adoption agencies and courts for mental health and economic stability had reduced the schizophrenia rate by over 60 percent.[73] Thus, in the beginning phases of their work the researchers uncovered—yet overlooked—important evidence suggesting that being reared in a more stable family environment reduced, by over one half, a child's chance of being diagnosed with schizophrenia later in life.[74]

The Arbitrary Inclusion of B3 "Borderline Schizophrenia" in the Spectrum

The investigators concluded that the Kety-led 1968 and 1975 results showed that "borderline schizophrenia" (B3) was genetically related to chronic schizophrenia, because it was significantly concentrated in the index biological relative group compared with the control group. However, they used improper methods of counting and combining diagnoses to arrive at this conclusion. For example, they counted the B3 biological relatives of B3 adoptees as evidence that B3 is genetically related to B1. As I showed in Chapter 3 of *The Missing Gene*, an examination of their results, based on proper methods of counting, leads to the opposite conclusion.[75]

Combining, Including, and Excluding Diagnostic Groups

One aspect of p-hacked research is investigators' post-data-analysis ability to combine or separate various categories to arrive at desired conclusions. I will cite a passage from a 1972 Rosenthal publication, and another from a 1988 Kety publication, to show how this occurred in the Danish-American adoption studies. In his 1972 article, Rosenthal wrote:

> The significant difference found in Table 6.1 was based primarily on the less severe forms of schizophrenic disorders, especially those called borderline or questionably borderline, and a subpsychotic form of disorder for which we do not have a really satisfactory name, which we have simply designated by the letter C. These combined diagnoses occurred about six times more frequently among the biological relatives of our index cases than among the biological relatives of the controls. *For this reason* [italics added] we feel justified in having broadened the range of schizophrenic disorders studied to include those that we thought might be genetically related to process [B1] schizophrenia. In this regard too, it is important to point out that the type of disorder that has been called reactive schizophrenia [B2] in the United States may have to be *excluded* [italics added] from the spectrum. Among the 30 biological relatives of 7 index cases who had this diagnosis, we did not find a single instance of schizophrenic spectrum disorder.[76]

The above passage captures the after-the-fact self-fulfilling prophecy that characterized the Danish-American adoption studies. The investigators found that certain spectrum diagnoses fell in ways that supported genetic assumptions, and "for this reason" they decided to include them. Other diagnoses, such as B2, did not support genetic assumptions, and for this reason they decided to exclude them. This practice made it likely that the researchers would arrive at conclusions in favor of genetics, since they constructed their schizophrenia spectrum as they went along to produce such conclusions.

In their 1988 report on the still-in-progress Provincial Study results, Kety and Loring Ingraham wrote:

> At the prototypical end of the spectrum, chronic schizophrenia is found exclusively in the biological relatives of chronic schizophrenia patients where it occurs at a low prevalence (approximately 3%), whereas the

prevalence in the biological relatives in the normal controls is negligible. The same is true for uncertain chronic schizophrenia. Latent or borderline schizophrenia was found at a 4-5% prevalence in the biological index relatives and 1% to 1.5% in the biological relatives of controls. This is also true where the symptoms are less distinct and the diagnosis is designated uncertain. *Since neither in chronic nor in latent schizophrenia the results for the definite or uncertain diagnoses are statistically different, it appears justified to combine them* [italics added].[77]

According to Kety, to achieve statistically significant findings it appeared "justified"—after the fact—to combine spectrum disorders in his study's statistical comparisons. However, he could have concluded that "since neither in chronic nor in latent schizophrenia the results for the definite or uncertain diagnoses are statistically different," the Provincial Study found no evidence that either chronic schizophrenia or latent schizophrenia was influenced by heredity. "Common practices that lead to p-hacking," wrote Megan Head and colleagues in 2015, "include ... combining, or splitting treatment groups postanalysis."[78]

Category C

The researchers based their 1968 Category C "inadequate personality" spectrum diagnosis on the 1968 DSM-II description. In the 1975 study, Category C was called "schizoid or inadequate personality." This diagnosis was not included in the 1980 DSM-III and subsequent editions. The complete DSM-II description of inadequate personality reads as follows:

> This behavior pattern is characterized by ineffectual responses to emotional, social, intellectual and physical demands. While the patient seems neither physically nor mentally deficient, he does manifest inadaptability, ineptness, poor judgement, social instability, and lack of physical and emotional stamina.[79]

In their 1968 and 1975 statistical calculations, Kety and colleagues counted relatives falling into this vague and non-psychotic category as having a schizophrenia spectrum disorder, a practice few mainstream authors have commented upon or criticized.

"Uncertain" Diagnoses in the Kety-led
Copenhagen Study (D1, D2, and D3)

"Uncertain" diagnoses (D1, D2, and D3) were counted as schizophrenia in the Danish-American adoption studies, including the triply vague "uncertain borderline schizophrenia" (D3) diagnosis. If the schizophrenia concept during this era was, as Thomas Szasz put it, "wonderfully vague in its content,"[80] then "borderline schizophrenia" was a questionable version of a vague diagnosis, and "uncertain borderline schizophrenia" was an uncertain version of a questionable version of a vague diagnosis.

In the 1975 Kety-led study, "uncertain" diagnoses represented 35 percent (13/37) of all index biological relative spectrum diagnoses, and an additional 35 percent were diagnosed Category C. *Together, these "uncertain" and "inadequate personality" diagnoses accounted for 70% (26/37) of all index biological relative schizophrenia spectrum diagnoses.*[81] The Kety-led studies helped inspire the initiation of molecular genetic research, but molecular genetic researchers have defined schizophrenia very differently from the studies that inspired them.

Diagnoses Based in Part on Sexual Orientation

As we have seen, the researchers' decision to include "borderline," "uncertain," and "inadequate personality" cases helped keep the study on track in the genetic direction. Their decision to include matters of sexual orientation and behavior provides a further example of their straying far from psychiatric conceptions of schizophrenia, and reflected the social and psychiatric prejudices of the era. (The APA removed, by vote, non-distressed homosexuality from its list of mental disorders in 1974.)

For Kety, Rosenthal, Wender, and colleagues, being judged as a "pervert,"[82] or as being "perverse (homosexual, transvestite)" was enough to land a person in their schizophrenia spectrum.[83] These researchers referred to same-sex sexual behavior or orientation as a symptom of schizophrenia in all three of their original 1968 "definite schizophrenia" diagnoses (see Table 6.2). Kety and colleagues' B1 diagnosis was characterized by "few heterosexual contacts," B2 included "homosexual panic," and B3 included a "mixture of hetero- and homosexuality."[84] Although they based these diagnoses on 1968 DSM-II diagnostic descriptions, the DSM-II did not mention anything about sexual orientation or behavior in its descriptions of the various types of schizophrenia.[85]

Having explored problems with the Danish-American schizophrenia spectrum concept, I will now discuss additional problems related specifically to the Kety-led studies and the Rosenthal-led study. I will examine only a few key areas, and I will continue to frame the analysis in the context of the many QRPs found in these studies.

Major Problem Areas in the Kety-led Copenhagen Study (1968–1975)

Changing the Research Design After the Results Came In

In this section I will provide evidence that Kety, Rosenthal, Wender, and colleagues abandoned their planned group comparison when they realized that it did not produce statistically significant results in the genetic direction, in favor of a different comparison that produced such results. My purpose here is to show how and why the researchers appear to have changed their group comparisons, not to speculate about which group comparisons they should have made.

In their 1968 publication, Kety and colleagues concluded in favor of genetics based on finding a significantly higher rate of spectrum diagnoses in the index biological (IB) versus the control biological (CB) relative groups:

> Of 150 biological relatives of index cases [IB], 13, or 8.7%, had a diagnosis of schizophrenia, uncertain schizophrenia or inadequate personality compared to 3 of 156, or 1.9%, with such diagnoses among the biological relatives of the controls [CB]. The difference is highly significant (*p*, one sided probability from exact distribution = 0.0072.[86]

The four relative groups are seen in Figure 6.3, which displays a simplified version of the relative groups shown in Figure 6.1.

In his 1959 *Science* article, however, Kety had envisioned an adoption study based on a different group comparison, one which would compare schizophrenia rates among the biological (IB) and adoptive (IA) relatives of adopted children later diagnosed with schizophrenia. As Kety wrote in this 1959 article:

> Another possible means of better controlling the environmental variables would be to make a careful study of schizophrenia in adopted children, with comparison of the incidence in blood relatives [IB] and in foster relatives [IA]. Perhaps only a survey on a national scale would provide the requisite numbers of cases for any of these studies.[87]

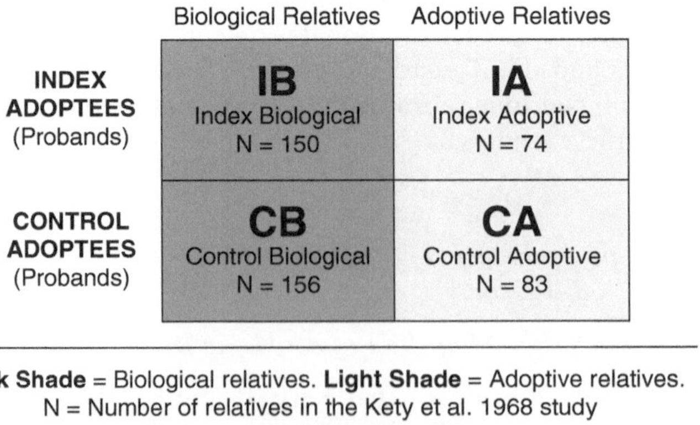

	Biological Relatives	Adoptive Relatives
INDEX ADOPTEES (Probands)	**IB** Index Biological N = 150	**IA** Index Adoptive N = 74
CONTROL ADOPTEES (Probands)	**CB** Control Biological N = 156	**CA** Control Adoptive N = 83

Dark Shade = Biological relatives. **Light Shade** = Adoptive relatives.
N = Number of relatives in the Kety et al. 1968 study

Figure 6.3 The Four Relative Groups in the Kety-led Studies

In a 1967 publication, which was based on a paper he presented at the March 29–31, 1967, First Rochester International Conference on Schizophrenia, Rosenthal described a planned comparison similar to Kety's 1959 *Science* description:

> In Denmark, with the collaboration of Dr. Fini Schulsinger and others, we began with adoptees who are now schizophrenic. We compare the incidence of schizophrenic disorders in their biological [IB] and adoptive [IA] families. The same procedure is carried out for a matched group of normal adoptees [CB versus CA], who serve as controls.[88]

Rosenthal was therefore on record as stating, as late as March 1967, that he and his colleagues intended to compare group IB versus IA relatives, and to then compare groups CB versus CA (control adoptive) relatives (see Figure 6.3). However, they did not begin their analyses of the data until April of 1967.[89] Apart from the above-quoted Kety and Rosenthal publications, I am not aware of any published or unpublished description of the Kety-led study's planned methods and group comparisons appearing prior to 1968.

The 1968 Kety-led study counted 13 schizophrenia spectrum disorders among the 150 IB relatives (8.7%) and 2 such disorders among the 74 IA relatives (2.7%).[90] As seen in Figure 6.4 the IB versus IA comparison was not statistically significant, meaning that if the researchers had stayed with their planned IB versus IA comparison, they would have had to conclude that their study found no evidence in favor of genetic influences on schizophrenia. Only through their decision to expand the definition of schizophrenia "as widely as it may have ever been reasonably conceived before," and to abandon their planned group comparisons, could they avoid reaching this conclusion.

Based on their new IB versus CB comparison, Kety and colleagues presented their findings to their colleagues at the Second Research Conference of the Foundations' Fund for Research in Psychiatry. This pivotal conference was attended by some of the world's leading schizophrenia researchers, including several leading psychiatric geneticists, and was held at Dorado Beach, Puerto Rico, between June 26 and July 1, 1967. Kety and colleagues published these findings the following year in *The Transmission of Schizophrenia*, a book containing papers presented at the conference. They *now* wrote in relation to the IB versus IA comparison, "Biological and adoptive parents differ in age, socio-economic class and in the particular selection process inherent in their having become biological or adoptive parents, making comparisons difficult between them with respect to the prevalence of mental illness." They mentioned these differences to justify basing their conclusions on the IB-CB comparison—a comparison they implied had been intended all along—where "none of these differences exist between the families of index cases and controls."[91]

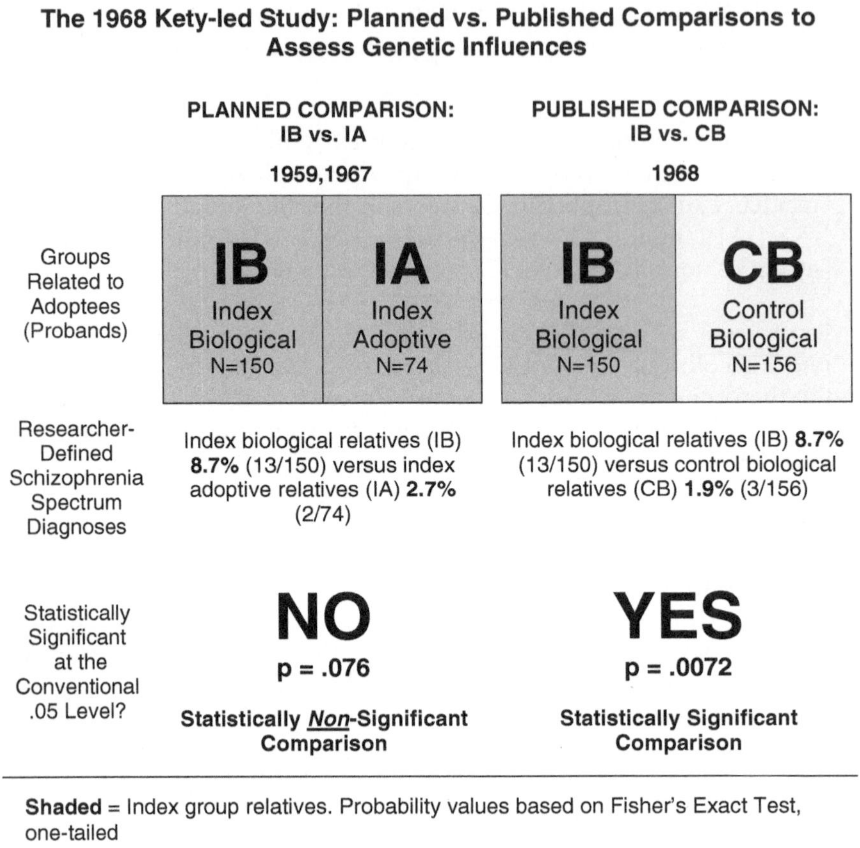

The 1968 Kety-led Study: Planned vs. Published Comparisons to Assess Genetic Influences

	PLANNED COMPARISON: IB vs. IA 1959, 1967		PUBLISHED COMPARISON: IB vs. CB 1968	
Groups Related to Adoptees (Probands)	**IB** Index Biological N=150	**IA** Index Adoptive N=74	**IB** Index Biological N=150	**CB** Control Biological N=156
Researcher-Defined Schizophrenia Spectrum Diagnoses	Index biological relatives (IB) **8.7%** (13/150) versus index adoptive relatives (IA) **2.7%** (2/74)		Index biological relatives (IB) **8.7%** (13/150) versus control biological relatives (CB) **1.9%** (3/156)	
Statistically Significant at the Conventional .05 Level?	**NO** p = .076 Statistically *Non*-Significant Comparison		**YES** p = .0072 Statistically Significant Comparison	

Shaded = Index group relatives. Probability values based on Fisher's Exact Test, one-tailed

Figure 6.4 The 1968 Kety-led Study: Planned versus Published Comparisons

LIDZ AND BLATT

Theodore Lidz and Sidney Blatt wrote in the April 1983 edition of the *American Journal of Psychiatry*, correctly as we have seen, that the "original purpose" of the Kety-led study had been "to differentiate genetic from intra-familial environmental factors by comparing the occurrence of disorders in the biological [IB] and adoptive [IA] relatives of schizophrenic patients who had been adopted at a very early age."[92] Theodore Lidz (1910–2001) was a psychodynamic psychiatrist and honored Yale University professor interested in the role of family environment in causing schizophrenia, and was the lead author of the 1965 book *Schizophrenia and the Family*.[93] Sidney Blatt (1928–2014) was a Yale psychologist interested in personality development. Lidz attended the March 1967 Rochester New York schizophrenia conference, and likely heard Rosenthal's talk describing the Kety-led study plan to test genetic theories based on the IB-IA comparison.[94]

Lidz was among the few psychiatry insiders who pointed to the glaring errors, biases, and manipulations in the Danish-American studies, but his views were marginalized by mainstream psychiatry at a time when the field was attempting to establish itself on DSM-III medical model principles amid a rhetorical "biological revolution in psychiatry." The medical model was celebrated in Nancy Andreasen's 1984 book *The Broken Brain*, where she asserted that the major psychiatric disorders "are ... diseases caused principally by biological factors, and most of these factors reside in the brain."[95]

Mainstream psychiatry saw Lidz and Blatt's critique as undermining its increasing emphasis on biology and genetics, and it took nearly 5 years for their unwelcomed manuscript to be published in the *American Journal of Psychiatry*. The article was first received by the *AJP* Editor in November 1978. After four revisions, it was accepted for publication in March of 1982, and finally appeared in print 13 months later in the April 1983 edition of the *Journal*. (This was well before the Internet era of pdfs, prepublication, and online journals.)[96] Although Lidz had been a major player in American psychiatry and had studied under Adolf Meyer, an influential leader of American psychiatry in the first half of the 20th century, he was now seen by ascendent biological psychiatry as a holdover from the environmentalist old guard unwilling to get on board the biological psychiatry train. The remaining clout he had, coupled with his perseverance, finally got his critique published in this top psychiatry journal.

KETY'S 1983 POSITION

In the June 1983 edition of the *American Journal of Psychiatry*, Kety responded to Lidz and Blatt's 1983 comment that his original intention had been to compare diagnoses among IB and IA relatives. Kety wrote that this objective "was not ours," and that "Lidz and Blatt have misunderstood 'the original purpose of the project' and the logic of our design." He denied that he and his colleagues had planned to make such a comparison, even though the Kety 1959 and Rosenthal 1967 publications clearly showed that they had.[97]

In a second 1983 response to Lidz and Blatt, in the form of a letter to the *American Journal of Psychiatry*, Kety again denied that he and his colleagues had ever made the IB-IA comparison or had "compute[d] its significance" before Lidz and Blatt raised the issue in 1983, because such a comparison would have been "improper" and "fallacious." As Kety wrote, "We did not make that comparison [IB versus IA], however, or compute its significance before this, because, for the reasons previously indicated... that comparison would have been improper and conclusions drawn from it fallacious."[98]

Kety's statement that "we did not make that comparison" prior to 1983 was false. As one example, in a 1974 *AJP* article, Kety made the IB-IA comparison, and said that the comparison was statistically significant in the genetic direction:

> For any of these diagnoses of schizophrenic illness, the prevalence in those genetically related to the schizophrenic index cases [IB] is 13.9 percent *compared to 2.7 percent in their adoptive relatives* [IA, italics added] or 3.8 percent in all subjects not genetically related to an index case [IA, CB, and CA]...These differences between the group genetically related to the schizophrenic index cases and those not so related *are highly significant statistically* [italics added] and speak for the operation of genetic factors in the transmission of schizophrenia.[99]

Kety decided to compute and publish the IB-IA comparison in 1974 because, after identifying additional relatives and conducting diagnostic interviews, the comparison was now statistically significant in the genetic direction. The evidence suggests that he and his colleagues had computed the IB-IA comparison seven years earlier in April/May 1967, but that they failed to publish or discuss this comparison because, at that earlier stage, the comparison *was not* statistically significant.

It appears that for Kety, with the results in hand, the planned IB versus IA comparison was "difficult," "improper," and "fallacious" when it failed to support the genetic position in 1967/1968, but spoke "for the operation of genetic factors" in 1974 when it appeared to him to support this position. Nine years later, Kety denied that he and his colleagues had ever planned or made IB-IA comparisons. QRP #6 identified by Leslie John and colleagues was at play here: "Selectively reporting studies that 'worked.'"

Overall, the evidence suggests that after viewing their 1967/1968 results, Kety and colleagues abandoned their planned IB-IA comparison when they saw that it failed to support genetic causation, in favor of the IB-CB comparison which they believed did support genetic causation, and then implied that the latter comparison had been planned all along. They arrived at genetic conclusions by HARKing ("hypothesizing after the results are known"), that is, they presented a *post*-data-analysis hypothesis as if it had been a *pre*-data-analysis hypothesis. As we saw in Chapter 1, the authors of the "Manifesto for Reproducible Science" concluded that HARKing "is not scientific discovery, but self-deception."[100]

Interviews and "Pseudointerviews" in the Kety-led 1975 Study

Substandard interviews were used to make diagnoses in the 1975 Kety-led study. Some of these "interviews" never took place, but instead were *fabricated by the investigators* based on hospital records. In the raw data Kety called these "pseudointerviews," but no mention of this practice appeared in any Danish-American publication I am aware of. According to Kendler and Gruenberg, who were given access to the raw data in the 1980s, "Based on an extensive review of hospital records, detailed pseudointerviews were constructed for all of the index adoptees."[101] Lewontin, Rose, and Kamin, the authors of *Not in Our Genes*, had been in correspondence with one of the psychiatrists conducting the interviews. According to these authors,

> In several cases, when relatives were dead or unavailable, the psychiatrist "prepared a so-called pseudo interview from the existing hospital records." That is, the psychiatrist filled out the interview form in the way in which he *guessed the relative would have answered.* [italics added].[102]

Psychologist David Jacobs (1945–2016) called this practice "outright fraud."[103] Of the interviews the researchers did conduct, they believed they could determine whether a reluctant, unfriendly, or hostile interviewee was in or out of the schizophrenia spectrum based on a five-minute doorstep conversation.[104]

No Significant Elevation of Schizophrenia in Either 1968 or 1975

The 1968 Kety-led study found *zero* cases of chronic schizophrenia (B1) among the 65 identified first-degree biological relatives of the index adoptee probands.[105] Had the researchers decided to count only these chronic cases—*as schizophrenia was defined in Denmark*—they would have concluded that they found no evidence that schizophrenia has a hereditary basis.[106] As Rosenthal subsequently admitted, "If we had relied only on hard-core, process [B1 chronic schizophrenia] cases, we would have found no significant difference between our index and control subjects."[107]

In the 1975 Kety-led study, the researchers reported a statistically significant B1 chronic schizophrenia rate among their index biological relatives (first- and second-degree) versus their control biological relatives. They counted five B1 diagnoses among these 173 index biological relatives, versus zero B1 diagnoses among the 174 control biological relatives. The index B1 rate was reported as statistically significant at the .03 level (5 vs. 0).[108] However, four of the five index biological relative diagnoses were given to half-siblings (two maternal, two paternal).[109]

It turns out that, even counting the half-siblings, the five index B1 biological relative diagnoses *did not* constitute a statistically significant clustering versus the control biological relatives. Kety and colleagues counted the biological father of control adoptee "C9" as B1 in 1968, but they decided not to count him as B1 in 1975 because he had died before he could be interviewed.[110] Had they continued to count his B1 diagnosis in 1975, the index-control difference would have been statistically *non*-significant (5 vs. 1).[111] Apparently, Kety and colleagues' 1975 evaluation of the biological father of control adoptee C9, and their decision to reverse his 1968 B1 diagnosis, was based on his "pseudointerview."

In 1988 Kety restored control adoptee C9's biological father as a Copenhagen B1 relative, but by then his diagnosis could be added to the Provincial Study totals, and the B1 comparison remained statistically significant.[112] Kety's decision to count C9's biological father as B1 in 1968, then to not count him as B1 in 1975, and to again count him as B1 in 1988 is a clear example of John and colleagues' QRP #7: "Deciding whether to exclude data after looking at the impact of doing so on the results."

High Rate of Spectrum Diagnoses Among Control Biological Relatives

The 1975 Kety-led study reported an 11 percent schizophrenia spectrum disorder rate (19/174) among all *control* biological relatives.[113] Based on a rough schizophrenia prevalence of 1 percent, by chance we would have expected only 1 or 2 of these 174 biological relatives of non-diagnosed control adoptees to have been diagnosed with schizophrenia. Kety and colleagues, however, expanded the definition of schizophrenia so widely that they produced a 10–15-fold increase of "schizophrenia" in the 1975 study. It's almost as if Kety singlehandedly created a mid-1970s schizophrenia epidemic in the city of Copenhagen.

Assumption Violation

In the Kety-led studies, psychologist Lorna Benjamin noted in 1976 that the "procedure of counting up all the possible relatives of each index case and pooling them as if they were independent samples . . . would allow some families to disproportionately affect the results."[114] Although Kety and colleagues did address this issue, their decision to emphasize the diagnostic rate among individual *relatives*, as opposed to individual *families*, violated the assumption of independent observations underlying the statistical methods they used. Because family environments may play a role in causing schizophrenia and psychosis, genetic study diagnoses given to people raised in the same family are not independent observations, for example, the Galvin sons and the Genain quadruplets.

In their 1975 publication, Kety and colleagues presented a table counting 14 index biological families as having one or more B1, B2, or B3 "definite schizophrenia" diagnosed members, versus 3 control families, a statistically significant difference.[115] However, as Lidz and Blatt, and later Boyle pointed out, Kety and colleagues miscounted the number of affected families as 14. The actual number was 8, a non-significant elevation.[116] For Boyle, it was "very difficult to understand how this mistake...was made in the first place." She noted that the error had "not been corrected," and that the incorrect figures continued to be cited.[117]

The "Compelling" Biological Paternal Half-Sibling Comparison Was Not Statistically Significant

We have seen that the Kety-led 1975 study found a significant concentration of spectrum disorders among the index (IB) versus control (CB) biological relatives. The researchers viewed this result as "compatible with a genetic transmission for schizophrenia, but it is not entirely conclusive."[118] Because of possible factors such as "*in utero* influences, birth trauma, and early mothering experiences," in the 1975 study Kety and colleagues wrote, appearing to negate their main 1968 and 1975 (and later 1994) conclusions, "One cannot, therefore, conclude that the high prevalence of schizophrenia illness found in these biological relatives of schizophrenics is genetic in origin."[119]

Kety and colleagues then made their case in 1975 for the discovery of "compelling evidence" in support of the "significant operation" of genetic factors, based on a comparison between the biological paternal half-siblings of their index and control adoptees. A biological paternal half-sibling is the offspring of an adoptee's biological father and a woman who is not the adoptee's biological mother. The adoptee and the half-sib did not grow up together and may not have known each other. Kety and colleagues described this group as follows:

> The largest group of relatives which we have is, understandably, the group of biological paternal half-siblings. Now, a biological paternal half-sibling of an index case has some interesting characteristics. He did not share the same uterus or the neonatal mothering experience, or an increased risk in birth trauma with the index case. The only thing they share is the same father and a certain amount of genetic overlap. Therefore, the distribution of schizophrenic illness in the biological paternal half-siblings is of great interest.[120]

The researchers counted 16 spectrum diagnoses among these paternal half-siblings, but found a "highly unbalanced" diagnostic distribution:14/63 index versus 2/64 control. They concluded, "We regard this as compelling evidence that genetic factors operate significantly in the transmission of schizophrenia."[121] Table 6.3 shows the paternal half-sibling results that Kety and colleagues presented in 1975 in support of their "compelling evidence" claim.

Lidz and Blatt made the point in 1983, however, that in the comparison seen in Table 6.3, *Kety and colleagues had to exclude schizophrenia-spectrum diagnosed relatives to find statistically significant results.* We

Table 6.3 Kety and Colleagues' 1975 Biological Paternal Half-Sibling Comparison[122]

Adoptees	Number of Biological Paternal Half-Siblings	Number Diagnosed "Definite"	Number Diagnosed "Uncertain"	TOTAL
Index (33)	63	8 (12.7%)	6 (9.5%)	14 (22.2%)
Control (34)	64	1 (1.6%)	1 (1.6%)	2 (3.1%)
		$p = .015$	$p = .055$	$p = .001$ Highly significant difference

p = one-tailed probability. Includes record- and interview-based diagnoses. All probability calculations by Kety et al. "Definite schizophrenia" diagnoses = B1+ B2 + B3; "Uncertain schizophrenia" diagnoses = D1 + D2 + D3

have already seen that in the 1968 and 1975 Kety-led studies, and in the Rosenthal-led studies, the investigators counted "schizoid or inadequate personality" (Category C) as a schizophrenia spectrum disorder.[123] To find statistically significant results, they decided to *remove* schizophrenia spectrum Category C-diagnosed biological paternal half-siblings from their 1975 comparison. The index versus control spectrum diagnosis difference was not statistically significant (p = .094) *when schizophrenia spectrum Category C is included.*[124] This is seen in Table 6.4

Kety and colleagues used Category C as their wild-card diagnosis. In 1968 and 1975 they played it in their relative groups to obtain more spectrum diagnoses, and then *temporarily* discarded it in the 1975 biological paternal half-sibling comparison because playing it there would have produced a statistically *non*-significant comparison. They played it again in the Provincial Study, and the schizoid/inadequate personality diagnosis remained in the spectrum until Kety decided to remove it in 1994 (see Table 6.5 below). Once again, open p-hacking, while better than hidden p-hacking, is still p-hacking.

As we saw in Chapter 1, the "scientific process requires that hypothesis development and hypothesis testing be based on *different* data sets. One data set is used to develop the hypothesis or model, which is used to make predictions, which are then tested on a new data set."[131] In 2020, Flint and colleagues emphasized this general point from a different angle: "*You cannot judge the probability of something happening after it's already happened.* In the literature this is called 'HARKing': Hypothesizing After the Result is Known."[132]

At most, Kety should have concluded in 1975 that the biological paternal half-sibling results provided an interesting exploratory finding that could be tested in a future study. It turns out that in the 1994 Provincial Study, the index versus control biological paternal half-sibling comparison again failed to reach statistical significance, even though Kety said that it did.[133]

Table 6.4 Kety and Colleagues' 1975 Biological Paternal Half-Sibling Comparison Including Schizophrenia Spectrum Category C[125]

Adoptees	Number of Biological Paternal Half-Siblings	Number Diagnosed "Definite"	Number Diagnosed "Uncertain"	NUMBER DIAGNOSED CATEGORY C	TOTAL
Index (33)	63	8 (12.7%)	6 (9.5%)	4 (6.3%)	18 (28.5%)
Control (34)	64	1 (1.6%)	1 (1.6%)	9 (14.1%)	11 (17.2%)
		p = .015	p = .055	--	p = .094
					Not statistically significant at the .05 level

p = one-tailed probability. All probability calculations by Kety et al. Includes record- and interview-based diagnoses. According to Kety and colleagues, "Definite schizophrenia" diagnoses = B1+ B2 + B3; "Uncertain schizophrenia" diagnoses = D1 + D2 + D3; Category C = schizophrenia spectrum "schizoid inadequate personality"

Major Problem Areas in the Kety-led Provincial Study (1978–1994)

Shifting Definitions of Schizophrenia

In the Kety-led Provincial Study, carried out in "the rest of Denmark" after completion of the Copenhagen study, the researchers retained and dropped diagnoses as they went along, over a 19-year period. The preliminary Provincial Study findings, based on records, were first published in 1978. The final interview-based Provincial Study publication appeared in 1994. Here I will briefly examine how the researchers defined and re-defined the spectrum during this 16-year period. Table 6.5 shows the researchers' shifting definition of the schizophrenia spectrum between 1978 and 1994.

Table 6.5 Shifting Components of the Danish-American Schizophrenia Spectrum: The Kety-led Provincial Study 1978–1994

1978: "Chronic schizophrenia," "Latent schizophrenia," "Acute schizophrenia," "Uncertain schizophrenia," "Schizoid personality"[126]

1985: "Chronic schizophrenia," "Latent schizophrenia," "Acute schizophrenia," "Uncertain schizophrenia," "Schizoid/inadequate personality"[127]

1988: "Certain and uncertain chronic schizophrenia," "Certain and uncertain latent schizophrenia," "Certain and uncertain acute schizophrenia," "Schizoid/inadequate personality disorder"[128]

1992: "Chronic schizophrenia," "Latent schizophrenia," "Schizoid personality"[129]

1994: "Chronic schizophrenia," "Latent schizophrenia"[130]

The Provincial Study began in 1975. In a 1978 publication, Kety, Rosenthal, Wender and colleagues defined the Provincial spectrum as consisting of "chronic schizophrenia," "latent schizophrenia," "acute schizophrenia," "uncertain schizophrenia," and "schizoid personality."[134] The Danish members of the team began interviewing Provincial relatives in 1980. In 1983 Kety wrote that, based on the 1975 Copenhagen results, Category C "schizoid and inadequate personality" relatives were "excluded from subsequent analyses" because "there was no...justification for believing that [these diagnoses]...were related to schizophrenia."[135] Then-recent research, Kety argued in 1983, supported the position that "schizoid or inadequate personality are not schizophrenia related."[136]

In a 1985 publication, however, Kety defined the spectrum as consisting of "chronic, latent, acute, and uncertain schizophrenia schizoid and inadequate personality as described in DSM-II."[137] In 1988, Kety again counted Provincial Study relatives diagnosed with one of these conditions as falling within the schizophrenia spectrum.[138] In other words, Kety continued to count the inadequate personality/schizoid diagnosis as a spectrum disorder five years after he had concluded, in American psychiatry's leading journal, that this diagnosis *did not* belong in the spectrum because it was "not schizophrenia related."

In 1992, *fourteen years* after the publication of the Provincial Study preliminary results, Kety decided to narrow the definition of the schizophrenia spectrum, describing this step more as something that happened as opposed to something he decided to do:

> Certain minor modifications evolved in our criteria or in their use between the Copenhagen and the Provincial studies. These included a decreased utilization of the DSM-II diagnoses "acute schizophrenia" or "pseudoneurotic schizophrenia," probably because of their lack of association with schizophrenia in the earlier study, and a recognition that "chronic" and "latent" schizophrenia were distinguishable whereas the gradations between "definite," "uncertain," or "probable" were not.[139]

In this passage Kety wrote of "minor modifications" of spectrum criteria that had "evolved" between the Copenhagen and Provincial Studies—as if researcher decision-making and hidden flexibility had played only a minor role in this "evolution." Had Kety chosen to describe this process clearly, he would have written that he and his colleagues, with the results in hand and over 14 years into the study, decided to perform a *major* modification of the spectrum by removing the "acute," "uncertain," and "probable" diagnoses.

In the final 1994 Provincial Study publication, Kety defined the spectrum as consisting only of "chronic schizophrenia" and "latent schizophrenia."[140] Kety's 1992/1994 decision to drop several spectrum categories while being aware of how they fell in his relative groups is an example of John and colleagues' QRP #1: "Failing to report all of a study's dependent measures."

Kety's Decision to Reduce the Size of the Provincial Study Index and Control Groups

In 1983, Kety reported that the Provincial Study proband groups consisted of 42 index and 42 control adoptees.[141] However, in the study's final 1994 publication, the adoptee proband groups consisted of only 33 index (29 chronic plus 4 latent) and 24 control adoptees. Kety did not clearly state in 1994 how and why he reduced his index adoptee proband group from 42 to 33, but it was probably due to his decision to remove the "acute" adoptee probands.

Turning to the control group, in 1994, almost two decades after the Provincial Study was initiated, Kety decided to remove 18 of his 42 control adoptee probands (43%) from the study. These included 13 interviewed control adoptees diagnosed with a "serious or confounding mental illness" (mainly non-spectrum affective disorders), plus 5 additional control adoptees on the grounds that they refused (or were unable) to be interviewed.[142] (In the 1975 Copenhagen Study, Kety decided to *retain* all 11 non-interviewed control adoptees.[143]) Kety's decision to remove these 18 control adoptee probands reduced the size of the control biological relative group from 178 to 121.[144] Kety did not disclose how many spectrum disorders were distributed among the 57 control biological relatives he removed from the study.

The Provincial Study and the 1994 Kendler et al. Analysis

Using data Kety supplied to them prior to the publication of the 1994 study, Kendler, Gruenberg, and Kinney published a 1994 "independent" review of the Kety et al. study in the same June 1994 edition of *Archives of General Psychiatry* (now *JAMA Psychiatry*). Kendler and colleagues' analysis was based on 42 index and 42 control adoptee probands found in Kety's unpublished data, even though we saw that the accompanying Kety et al. 1994 publication was based on only 33 index and 24 control adoptees. Prior to submitting their articles, the Kendler and Kety groups had been in communication after the first draft of each group's manuscript had been completed.[145]

The *Archives* accepted Kendler and colleagues' manuscript for publication on July 29, 1993,[146] and accepted Kety and colleagues' manuscript for publication on February 25, 1994.[147] Based on these dates, the evidence suggests that—19 years into the study—Kety decided to reduce the size of his Provincial Study's index group from 42 to 33 adoptee probands, and his control group from 42 to 24 adoptee probands, just as the evidence suggests that he and his colleagues had scrambled in the Spring of 1967 to make last-minute group comparison changes prior to presenting their Copenhagen results at Dorado Beach.

A 1993 article by Kendler and Scott Diehl reported that in the Provincial Study prepublication data, "latent and uncertain schizophrenia was not found to be significantly more common in the biologic relatives of the schizophrenia adoptees than in those of the control adoptees (6.5% vs. 5.5%, respectively)."[148] This might explain why Kety decided to remove latent and uncertain schizophrenia from the spectrum prior to publishing the 1994 final report. John and colleagues QRPs #1 and #7 apply here: "Failing to report all of a study's dependent measures," and "Deciding whether to exclude data after looking at the impact of doing so on the results."

Other Problem Areas

Additional problem areas in the Kety-led 1994 Provincial Study's attempt to "replicate" the earlier Copenhagen results in the rest of Denmark include the following points: (1) The study was subject to most of the problems and biases found in the 1968 and 1975 studies, and like these earlier studies there was selective placement bias in the sample. (2) In Kendler and colleagues' above-mentioned 1994 analysis based on DSM-III diagnostic criteria, the chronic schizophrenia rate among all index biological relatives of adoptees with the same diagnosis was 2.3 percent (2/88). This rate was not significantly higher than the control biological relative rate of .6 percent (1/162), or versus the general population expectation.[149] This comparison remained statistically non-significant when limited to first-degree relatives.[150] (3) There was no statistically significant first-degree biological relative index group elevation of "latent schizophrenia" when compared with controls.[151] (4) The symptoms of "latent schizophrenia" were vague, and were often indistinguishable from non-spectrum psychiatric diagnoses.[152] (5) The researchers counted a total of 3 diagnoses of "chronic schizophrenia" among the 24 first-degree biological full-siblings of the 29 index adoptees with the same diagnosis. However, all three were members of the same family,[153] suggesting that family environment, rather than genetic background, best explains this clustering of chronic schizophrenia among siblings reared together in the same family—again, just as it did in the Galvin and Genain families.

As opposed to the usual textbook claim that the Provincial Study replicated the Copenhagen genetic findings, it instead replicated the biases, QRP data manipulation and p-hacking, and the failure to recognize the impact of environmental confounds that characterized the earlier Copenhagen work.

Major Problem Areas in the Rosenthal-led Study (1968–1978)

No Evidence in Support of Genetics in 1968

The 1968 Rosenthal-led study publication reported that only 1 of the 39 adopted-away biological offspring of a parent diagnosed with a schizophrenia spectrum disorder had received a hospital diagnosis of chronic (B1) schizophrenia.[154] Rosenthal, Kety, Wender and colleagues could simply have stopped at this point and concluded that, despite several years of painstaking research across two continents, they found no evidence in favor of genetic influences on schizophrenia. Like the Kety-led studies, a great deal of remarkably out-in-the-open p-hacking was necessary to transform negative genetic results to positive ones.

Discussing their 1968 findings, Rosenthal and colleagues wrote:

> One inference ought to be drawn from this data: that is, if we are going to learn anything more about the genetics of schizophrenic disorders, we can no longer rely on statistics based only on hospitalized cases. Had we done so in this study, we would have concluded that heredity did not

contribute significantly to schizophrenia, or that, if it did, the gene was probably recessive.[155]

My translation of Rosenthal's description of researcher behavior now known as p-hacking: *Our planned study found no evidence that heredity plays a role in causing schizophrenia. Instead of ending our study with that conclusion, our genetic confirmation biases compelled us to keep looking for more cases in support of psychiatric genetic assumptions and theories.* For Rosenthal, Kety, Wender and colleagues, a conclusion that "heredity did not contribute significantly to schizophrenia" was not an acceptable conclusion. They reasoned that if the results showed no evidence of genetic causes, there must be something wrong with the data, or with the study design, that needed to be fixed.

Collecting Cases Past the 1968 Data-Collection Stop Point

Despite using a very broad definition of schizophrenia, Rosenthal and colleagues claimed no statistically significant findings in their 1968 study. However, they stressed that their results were "preliminary" and that "the N is small and will increase considerably."[156] "The figures presented today are not final," they wrote. "We are still collecting subjects," and "the patterns we have seen so far could change."[157] "The story we hope to tell has only begun to unfold."[158] In his 1971 book *Genetics of Psychopathology*, Rosenthal said that "the study is still in progress."[159] Clearly, in 1968 Rosenthal saw his findings as "preliminary" and in need of more participants only because these findings did not support his "diathesis-stress" theory of schizophrenia.

Because the study's planned data-collection stop-point, assuming there was one, was known only to the researchers (hidden flexibility), Rosenthal and colleagues continued adding parent probands after 1968 with the hope of finding enough diagnoses among their adopted-away offspring to be able to tell "the story we hope to tell"—a tactic apparently acceptable at the time, but now properly regarded as a classic p-hacking maneuver. Rosenthal and colleagues had the additional hidden option of stopping the study exactly at the point at which the comparison dipped below the .05 level of statistical significance, as they apparently did in their study's 1971 publication, again in classic p-hacking fashion. "The story we hope to tell has only begun to unfold" is another way of saying, *we refuse to accept the negative results of the scientific experiment we just conducted.*

Questionable research practices of this type can occur when researchers are not required to adhere to a stated data-collection stop point, which would be established and documented in a preregistered study. We have seen that in a different context, psychologist Stuart Ritchie noted that "not setting the sample size beforehand allows...researchers to continue collecting data and testing it, collecting data and testing it, again and again in an open-ended way until they get their desired p < 0.05."[160] This describes to a tee the p-hacking strategy Rosenthal employed in his study.

Counting "Manic-Depression" as a Schizophrenia Spectrum Disorder

In the Rosenthal-led studies (but not in the Kety-led studies), the researchers counted "manic-depression" as a schizophrenia spectrum disorder,[161] despite Rosenthal's belief that schizophrenia and manic-depression are "genetically distinct and different disorders."[162] Without these manic-depressive cases, Rosenthal and colleagues would not have been able to claim statistically significant results in the genetic direction in their 1971 publication.[163]

Even though Rosenthal viewed schizophrenia and manic-depression (now known as bipolar disorder) as genetically distinct and different disorders, the 1971 Rosenthal-led study listed "manic-depressive psychosis" as one of the diagnoses "that we are tentatively including in the 'schizophrenia spectrum.'"[164] Five years later Rosenthal, Kety and colleagues claimed, falsely, that "manic-depressive illness was never thought to be in the schizophrenia spectrum by us."[165]

The researchers agreed to diagnose 7 of the 76 (9%) index biological parent probands with manic-depressive disorder in 1971, and at least one of them diagnosed an additional 17 parents (22%) with this condition.[166] Why did parents diagnosed with this "genetically distinct and different disorder" qualify them as a schizophrenia index parent proband? Rosenthal offered two explanations in 1968:

> These [manic-depressive] cases were included for two reasons. The first was one of expediency. There were periods when we simply did not have enough schizophrenic parents processed and the staff in Copenhagen had no subjects to examine. The second and more important reason derived from this question: What if we should find differences between our Index and Control groups. . . . If we had a comparison pathology group, we might be able to learn something. . . . about the possible genetic relationship between schizophrenia and manic-depressive psychosis.[167]

Rosenthal thereby included an admittedly non-related diagnosis in a schizophrenia genetic study for reasons of "expediency." Imagine the folly of a study on the genetics of heart disease that added liver disease patients because the staff "had no heart disease subjects to examine," and then decided to count liver disease as a "heart disease spectrum disorder." Turning to the second reason, the use of an unrelated diagnosis to create a "comparison pathology group" does not mean that the diagnosis should be counted as belonging to the group it is being compared with, which Rosenthal decided to do. In the words of psychologist Alvin Pam, a critic of this study, the inclusion of manic-depressive parents rendered the study "invalid on its face."[168] Lidz and colleagues argued that "the study could no longer properly be termed a study of adopted-away offspring of schizophrenic parents."[169] Indeed, it couldn't.

Final Result of the Rosenthal-led Study: Negative

As we have seen, in the 1968 and 1971 Rosenthal-led studies the researchers did not arrive at consensus (global) diagnoses for their index and control adoptees, but instead relied on what they called "thumbnail diagnostic formulations" prepared by Danish psychiatrist co-authors Joseph Welner and Fini Schulsinger.

In a 1978 article by Richard Haier, Rosenthal, and Wender, which to the best of my knowledge was the final Rosenthal-led study publication, the researchers reported their index and control group adoptee consensus schizophrenia spectrum diagnoses for the first and final time. The results showed no statistically significant difference between these two groups on the basis of a Haier, Rosenthal, and Wender-defined schizophrenia spectrum consisting of chronic schizophrenia, borderline schizophrenia, and "schizophrenic personality" (index 32% vs. control 26%).[170] Haier et al. reported these results in a table, but chose to discuss them only in the context of whether scores on the psychological test they administered (the Minnesota Multiphasic Personality Inventory, or MMPI) differentiated between the two groups. This enabled them to conclude that their findings "support the genetic hypothesis."[171]

The take-home point, however, is that based on the Rosenthal-led study's final definition of what counted as a schizophrenia spectrum disorder, there was no significant difference between the index and control adoptee groups. As Lewontin and colleagues correctly concluded in 1984, "despite the widely misleading early reports on the Rosenthal et al. study, its outcome was in fact negative."[172]

Summary of Questionable Research Practices Used in the Kety-led and Rosenthal-led Studies

Table 6.6 summarizes the QRPs used in the Kety-led and Rosenthal-led studies. These 10 QRPs were introduced in Chapter 1, and are taken from Leslie John and colleagues' 2012 survey of psychologists' use of QRPs.[173]

A major objective of this chapter has been to show that Kety, Rosenthal and colleagues needed to use multiple QRPs across multiple studies to achieve statistically significant results in the genetic direction. In the next section we will see that psychiatry and behavioral science publications usually tell a different story.

Table 6.6 Summary of Questionable Research Practices in the Danish-American Schizophrenia Adoption Studies[174]

Questionable Research Practice (QRP)	Kety-led Studies	Rosenthal-led Study
1. "Failing to report all of a study's dependent measures"	✔	✔
2. "Deciding whether to collect more data after looking to see whether the results were significant"		✔
3. "Failing to report all of a study's conditions"	✔	✔
4. "Stopping collecting data earlier than planned because one found the result that one had been looking for"		✔
5. "'Rounding off' a *p*-value (e.g., reporting that a *p*-value of .054 is less than .05)"		
6. "Selectively reporting studies that 'worked'"	✔	✔
7. "Deciding whether to exclude data after looking at the impact of doing so on the results"	✔	✔
8. "Reporting an unexpected finding as having been predicted from the start" (HARKing)	✔	✔
9. "Claiming that results are unaffected by demographic variables when one is actually unsure (or knows that they do)"	✔	✔
10. "Falsifying data"		

Misleading Accounts of Schizophrenia Adoption Research

Despite their massive flaws, the legend of the Danish-American adoption studies lives on because most contemporary researchers, clinicians, academics, and others learn about these studies from the authors of expert reviews and textbooks. Here I provide some examples of misleading and misinformed accounts often found in these writings.

In 2002, Jonathan Leo and I reviewed Nobel Prize–winning psychiatrist Eric Kandel's chapter on schizophrenia in the 2000 edition of *Principles of Neural Science*. We highlighted several errors and noted the genetic/biological bias in Kandel's discussion of schizophrenia research.[175] In Chapter 5 of *The Missing Gene* I documented major problems with psychiatry and abnormal psychology textbook accounts of schizophrenia adoption research. These problems included that their authors sometimes or often (1) emphasized the original researchers' conclusions at the expense of independent critical analysis; (2) relied on secondary sources; (3) failed to discuss, or mentioned only briefly, the views and publications of critics; (4) misreported studies' methods and results; (5) failed to discuss problems with the reliability and validity of a schizophrenia diagnosis in the context of genetic research; (6) failed to discuss potential adoption study environmental confounds such as prenatal environment, late separation, late placement, range restriction, and selective placement; (7) cited studies failing to find statistically significant results in the genetic direction as evidence in favor of genetics; and (8) accepted the original researchers' definition of schizophrenia without question, and used the word "schizophrenia" when discussing what in fact were Kety, Rosenthal, and Wender-defined "schizophrenia spectrum disorders." Unfortunately, little has changed since 2006.

I now provide additional examples of how the authors of important works misrepresented adoption studies' methods and results. These publications include leading textbooks in psychiatry: The APA's prestigious *American Psychiatric Publishing Textbook of Psychiatry*, edited by Robert Hales and colleagues, and the Kaplan and Sadock series.

Citing Nonexistent Reared-Apart (Adoptive) Twin Studies

We have seen that apart from a handful of anecdotal single-case reports I discussed briefly in Chapter 5, reared-*apart* schizophrenia twin studies, also known as "adoptive-twin studies," do not exist. Nevertheless, the 1996 edition of Kaplan and Sadock's *Concise Textbook of Clinical Psychiatry* contained the following description:

> Monozygotic twins have the highest concordance rate. The studies of adopted monozygotic twins show that twins who are reared by adoptive parents have schizophrenia at the same rate as their twin siblings raised by their biological parents. That finding suggests that the genetic influence outweighs the environmental influence.[176]

Kaplan and Sadock described studies using reared-apart MZ pairs, where one group consisted of MZ twins raised by their biological parents, while the other group consisted of their adopted-away (separated) MZ co-twins raised by their adoptive parents. They provided no references for such studies. Because, they said, these studies showed that both twin groups have the same schizophrenia rate, the "genetic influence outweighs the environmental influence." In fact, *no such studies exist.*

Misleading accounts are also found in Hales and colleagues' *American Psychiatric Publishing Textbook of Psychiatry*. In a passage found in the 2003 edition's "Genetics" chapter by James Knowles, which was repeated in the 2008 edition chapter by Prabhakara Choudary and Knowles, the authors reported that "two studies of MZ twins reared apart have shown high pairwise concordance for schizophrenia, providing further evidence for a genetic component in the etiology of this disorder."[177] Again, no reared-apart (adoptive) twin studies for schizophrenia exist.

The authors of a chapter on schizophrenia in the Hales-edited 2011 edition of *Essentials of Psychiatry* wrote, "Twin adoption studies have been remarkably consistent in reporting approximately 50% concordance rate [*sic*] for monozygotic twins."[178] This is the standard claim for studies of reared-*together* pairs, but we have seen that a "twin adoption" study is another name for a reared-apart twin study, which doesn't exist in psychiatry.

Incorrect Descriptions of the Comparison
Groups Used in the Kety-led Studies

Although we have seen that genetic conclusions in the Kety-led publications were based on comparisons between the index biological relative (IB) versus the control biological relative (CB) groups (see Figures 6.3 and 6.4), many subsequent commentators wrote incorrectly that Kety's research was based on IB versus index adoptee (IA) comparisons. Before citing examples of authors who got this wrong, I will cite an example of an author who got it right. In a 1988 textbook chapter, Kendler wrote,

> Another major adoption strategy used for studying schizophrenia begins with ill adoptees rather than with ill relatives…A comparison of the biological relatives of the two groups of adoptees [IB versus CB] is a test for the role of genes in the familial transmission of schizophrenia. This strategy has been used by Kety and colleagues in a series of adoption studies carried out in Denmark.[179]

We recall that in 1983, Kety stated that it would be "improper" and "fallacious" to compare spectrum diagnoses between the IB and IA groups. Earlier, in a 1976 publication, Kety and colleagues wrote, "Another type of inappropriate comparison that some have made is that between adoptive and biological relatives."[180] Nevertheless, many well-known authors have written, mistakenly, that genetic conclusions in the Kety-led studies were based on IB versus IA comparisons.

This error is seen even within one of Kety and colleagues' own publications. In a 1971 article in the *American Journal of Psychiatry* by Kety, Rosenthal, Wender, and Schulsinger describing the 1968 Kety-led study, the article's abstract said,

> In the study reported here, a significantly higher than usual prevalence of schizophrenia-related illness was found among the biological relatives of adopted schizophrenics [IB], but not among their adoptive relatives [IA]. The findings support a genetic transmission of vulnerability to schizophrenia… .[181]

In the main body of the article, however, the IB-CB comparison was used.

In his 2004 book *The Agile Gene: How Nature Turns on Nurture*, science writer Matt Ridley wrote that Kety "found that schizophrenia was 10 times as common in the biological relatives of diagnosed schizophrenics who had been adopted as children as it was in their adopting families."[182] Additional mistaken claims that the Kety-led studies were based on IB-IA comparisons are found in the 2000 edition of *Kaplan & Sadock's Comprehensive Textbook of Psychiatry*, and in the 2008 edition of Kaplan and Sadock's *Concise Textbook of Clinical Psychiatry*.[183]

Similarly mistaken claims that the Kety-led studies' conclusions were based on IB versus IA comparisons are found in the publications of many of the world's leading psychiatric and psychiatric genetic researchers. Works in which this error was made include Ming Tsuang and Randall Vandermey's 1980 *Genes and the Mind*; a 1989 review article by James Kennedy, Kenneth Kidd, Luca Cavalli-Sforza, Hans Moises and colleagues; a 1991 chapter by Michael Lyons, Kenneth Kendler, Anne Gersony Provet, and Tsuang in *Genetic Issues in Psychosocial Epidemiology*; the 1994 book *Seminars in Psychiatric Genetics* by Peter McGuffin, Michael Owen, Michael O'Donovan, Anita Thapar, and Irving Gottesman; Jerrold Maxmen and Nicholas Ward's 1995 *Essential Psychopathology and Its Treatment*; Brien Riley, Philip Asherson, and McGuffin's chapter in the 2003 textbook *Schizophrenia*; the Alastair Cardno and McGuffin, and the Owen, O'Donovan, and Gottesman chapters in the 2003 book *Psychiatric Genetics and Genomics*; the 2003 Owen and O'Donovan chapter in *Behavioral Genetics in the Postgenomic Era*; a 2005 "Genetics of Schizophrenia" article by Patrick Sullivan; Rajiv Tandon and colleagues' 2008 "Schizophrenia, Just the Facts" article; and a 2012 chapter by Hugh Gurling and Andrew McQuillin in *Principles of Psychiatric Genetics*.[184] These expert psychiatric geneticists and their supporters have been telling us about the Kety-led studies for decades, but they do not appear to understand how Kety and colleagues arrived at their conclusions.

Lynn DeLisi, Robert Freedman, and Robert Kolker

In Chapter 3 I reviewed Robert Kolker's 2020 book *Hidden Valley Road*, the tragic story of an American family in which six of the ten male children were eventually diagnosed with schizophrenia, and three committed suicide. The featured molecular genetic investigators in this book were Lynn DeLisi and Robert Freedman. They and Kolker saw the publication of the Danish-American adoption studies as a major turning point in support of psychiatric genetic theories of schizophrenia, yet none appeared to understand the basic design of these studies.

In her 2017 popular work *100 Questions & Answers About Schizophrenia: Painful Minds*, DeLisi wrote incorrectly that in the Kety-led 1968 study, the "investigators showed that an excess of schizophrenia was present in the biological relatives of individuals with schizophrenia [IB], but not the adoptive relatives [IA]."[185] Like many authors, DeLisi said that the Danish-American studies counted diagnoses of "schizophrenia," when in fact they counted spectrum disorders ranging all the way down to "uncertain borderline schizophrenia," "inadequate personality," and "manic-depressive psychosis." In a 2022 publication, DeLisi continued to misrepresent and misunderstand how the Danish-American studies were performed.[186]

In his 2010 book *The Madness Within Us: Schizophrenia as a Neuronal Process*, Robert Freedman wrote that the "most dramatic proof that schizophrenia is a heritable illness" was provided by the Danish-American studies:

The demonstration that the risk for schizophrenia in children of mothers who have schizophrenia remains, even if the child is adopted by another mother close to the time of birth, was historically the most dramatic proof that schizophrenia is a heritable illness and hence a biologically based outcome, rather than a psychologically based outcome.[187]

This is a rough description of the Rosenthal-led study design. However, Freedman cited the previously discussed Kety et al. 1971 article, which described the Kety-led study.[188]

In Chapter 14 of *Hidden Valley Road*, Kolker's descriptions of the Danish-American adoption studies and the 1967 Dorado Beach Conference were inaccurate. To mention one example, Kolker said that the 1968 Kety-led study researchers "compared their adoptees to a control group—schizophrenia patients who grew up in their own families." This is not an accurate description.[189] Kolker wrote approvingly that at Dorado Beach, Rosenthal "discredited the idea that bad parenting created the [schizophrenia] disease."[190] I am not aware of Rosenthal making such a statement, and we saw that his 1968 study produced no statistically significant results in the genetic direction. Kolker was fully aware of the Genain Quadruplets' story, but apparently "bad parenting" had nothing to do with the quads' common descent into psychosis.[191]

Past President of the APA

Former APA President Jeffrey Lieberman wrote a 2016 op-ed piece in the *Wall Street Journal*, where he cited research that never took place in support of genetic theories of schizophrenia.[192] Lieberman is the author of over 600 papers and articles published in the scientific literature, and was the lead editor of the 2020 second edition of the *American Psychiatric Publishing Textbook of Schizophrenia*.[193]

Lieberman and co-author Ogi Ogas said that Kety's "data" produced a "genetic riddle," that the MZ co-twin of someone diagnosed with schizophrenia is "50% likely to develop the illness—not the 100% expected." Kety, however, did not study twins, nor did he publish any original schizophrenia twin data.

Again referring to "Kety's data," Lieberman and Ogas wrote that "if both your parents had schizophrenia, you were only 50 percent likely to develop the illness." Here they were apparently referring to the so-called "dual mating" studies of the offspring of two parents diagnosed with schizophrenia. The rates are lower than 50 percent, but the relevant point is that Kety never performed a dual mating study either.[194] In their 2015 book *Shrinks: The Untold Story of Psychiatry*, Lieberman and Ogas said that Kety "settled the question of schizophrenia's genetic basis" by finding a higher IB versus IA schizophrenia rate.[195] Not true.

Like Siddhartha Mukherjee (see Chapter 5), Lieberman appeared to be unfamiliar with the original "evidence" that psychiatry constantly puts forward as proof that its disorders are both valid and "heritable." Even more concerning is that this former APA president informed his readers of important findings produced by nonexistent studies. Lieberman, Mukherjee, and the other authors I mentioned did not intentionally present the facts incorrectly, but when one sees the genetic basis of schizophrenia as a proven fact, it doesn't seem necessary to carefully read, review, and understand the original research.

Does anyone other than persistent critics and a few other informed authors understand how the Danish-American schizophrenia adoption studies were performed, and how Kety, Rosenthal, Wender and colleagues arrived at their conclusions?

Summary and Conclusions

In this chapter I described the schizophrenia adoption studies and focused on the two most frequently cited: the Kety-led and Rosenthal-led Danish-American investigations. I described several potentially confounding aspects of psychiatric adoption research, including selective placement, late separation and late placement, range restriction and the screening of adoptive families, and shared pre-natal environment. I then closely examined the Kety-led and Rosenthal-led studies, and showed that their authors' conclusions in favor of genetic influences on schizophrenia are not supported by the findings. To arrive at these conclusions and to tell "the story we hope to tell," the evidence shows or strongly suggests that the Danish-American adoption researchers (1) denied any major impact of environmental confounds on their findings, (2) manipulated and greatly expanded (and then narrowed when necessary) the definition of schizophrenia, (3) kept looking for additional schizophrenia spectrum cases and called their study preliminary after finding statistically non-significant results, and (4) changed comparison groups when the planned group comparison failed to produce evidence in support of genetic causation. Finally, I highlighted misleading and uninformed accounts of these studies by influential authors and publications.

There are additional problems in the Danish-American studies that I chose not to cover in the interest of not lengthening an already lengthy chapter. Among these problems are the researchers' decision to count full- and half-siblings with equal genetic weighting, the questionable logic behind their decision to eventually remove B2 "acute schizophrenia" from the schizophrenia spectrum, the lack of case history information for adoptees and their families (John and colleagues' QRP #3), the use of late-separated adoptees, that diagnostic rates among index adoptees or relatives must significantly exceed the rate expected in the general population, problems with the interview process, additional examples of inconsistent methods of counting dead or unavailable relatives, counting "uncertain" relative diagnoses as schizophrenia for the purpose of preventing these relatives from becoming "lost,"[196] and differences between E. Bleuler's description of latent schizophrenia versus Kety and colleagues' descriptions of Bleuler's views.[197]

The basic story of the Danish-American schizophrenia adoption studies that future textbooks should tell is that, after several years of painstaking transatlantic research in the 1960s, the investigators found no evidence that schizophrenia was caused by hereditary factors. Instead of simply acknowledging this finding, and then publishing these negative results with little recognition, they decided to open up what Rosenthal called a "Pandora's box" by greatly expanding the definition of schizophrenia in an attempt to find results that confirmed their preexisting belief that genetic factors underlie schizophrenia.[198] As psychologist Richard Bentall concluded, "When Rosenthal and Kety were unable to find clear genetic effects with a conventional definition of schizophrenia they simply expanded their definition.... The spectrum concept was merely introduced so that the researchers could get the result they wanted."[199]

Generations of students, clinicians, "patients," researchers, and others have been misled through the process I described in Chapter 1: psychiatric genetic investigators produce unsound research based on false assumptions and/or manipulated or misinterpreted data → researchers producing this unsound research are rewarded, funded, and honored → respected academic fields endorse and promote this unsound research in textbooks and other publications → the media reports on and promotes this unsound research → the works of journalists and highly respected researchers and authors promote and celebrate unsound research → the academic world and the general public are convinced by the above process that what is in fact unsound research is actually sound research.

As Stephen Jay Gould showed in *The Mismeasure of Man*, human genetic research has a long history of investigators "shifting criteria to work through good data toward desired conclusions," and creating conditions in which "data" are not allowed to "overthrow ... assumptions."[200] As a careful examination of their published works reveals, the Danish-American researchers continued this unfortunate tradition—simply refusing to permit their data to overthrow psychiatry's need to establish "schizophrenia" as a valid genetic/biological medical disorder. In addition, for the reasons I discussed, the results of the Heston, Tienari, and Lichtenstein studies cannot be interpreted genetically.

The Danish-American schizophrenia adoption studies are perhaps the longest running example of p-hacked research ever seen in the behavioral sciences, and as such should not survive the replication crisis. As I have shown in this chapter, the evidence is "compelling" that these studies should be retracted. Textbooks should be rewritten to reflect these developments, and the Danish-American studies should be presented as a replication crisis case study of how *not* to do science.

Notes

1 An unnamed academic supervisor. Quoted in Chambers, C. (2017), *The Seven Deadly Sins of Psychology: A Manifesto for Reforming the Culture of Scientific Practice*, Princeton, NJ: Princeton University Press, p. 175.

2 My previous writings on schizophrenia adoption research include Joseph, J. (1998), *A Critical Analysis of the Genetic Theory of Schizophrenia*, unpublished doctoral dissertation, California School of Professional Psychology, Alameda; Joseph, J. (2001), The Danish-American Adoptees' Family Studies of Kety and Associates: Do They Provide Evidence in Support of the Genetic Basis of Schizophrenia?, *Genetic, Social, and General Psychology Monographs, 127*, 241–278; Joseph, J. (2004), *The Gene Illusion: Genetic Research in Psychiatry and Psychology Under the Microscope*, New York: Algora, Chapter 7; Joseph, J. (2006), *The Missing Gene: Psychiatry, Heredity, and the Fruitless Search for Genes*, New York: Algora, Chapter 3; Joseph, J. (2013), "Schizophrenia" and Heredity: Why the Emperor (Still) Has No Genes, in J. Read & J. Dillon (Eds.), *Models of Madness: Psychological, Social and Biological Approaches to Psychosis* (2nd ed.; pp. 72–89), London: Routledge.

3 Rosenthal, D. (1970), *Genetic Theory and Abnormal Behavior*, New York: McGraw-Hill, p. 56.

4 Cassou et al. (1980), Génétique et Schizophrénie: Réévaluation d'un Consensus [Genetics and Schizophrenia: Reevaluation of a Consensus], *Psychiatrie de l'Enfant*, 23, 87–201.

5 Newman et al. (2015), Attachment and Early Brain Development—Neuroprotective Interventions in Infant-Caregiver Therapy, *Translational Developmental Psychiatry*, 3: 28647. https://doi.org/10.3402/tdp.v3.28647; Shore, A. N. (2001), Effects of a Secure Attachment Relationship on Right Brain Development, Affect Regulation, and Infant Mental Health, *Infant Mental Health Journal, 22*, 7–66. https://doi.org/10.1002/1097-0355(200101/04)22:1<7::AID-IMHJ2>3.0.CO;2-N;

6 Sham, P. C., & Kendler, K. S. (2008), Genetic Etiology, in R. Murray et al. (Eds.), Essential Psychiatry (4th ed., pp. 80–94), Cambridge: Cambridge University Press, p. 85.

7 Heston, L. L. (1966), Psychiatric Disorders in Foster Home Reared Children of Schizophrenic Mothers, *British Journal of Psychiatry, 112*, 819–825. https://doi.org/10.1192/bjp.112.489.819

8 Heston, 1966, p. 823.

9 Heston, L. L. (1970), The Genetics of Schizophrenic and Schizoid Disease, *Science, 167*, 249–256. https://doi.org/10.1126/science.167.3916.249

10 Joseph, 2004.

11 Heston, L. L., & Denny, D. D. (1968), Interactions Between Early Life Experience and Biological Factors in Schizophrenia, in D. Rosenthal & S. Kety (Eds.), *The Transmission of Schizophrenia* (pp. 363–376), New York: Pergamon Press, p. 369; Heston, 1966, p. 822.

12 Heston & Denny, 1968, p. 374.

13 For more on Heston's study, see Joseph, 2004, pp. 204–212.

14 Kety, S. S. (1959), Biochemical Theories of Schizophrenia, Part II, *Science, 129*, 1590–1596. https://doi.org/10.1126/science.129.3363.1590

15 Kety et al. (1978), The Biologic and Adoptive Families of Adopted Individuals Who Became Schizophrenic: Prevalence of Mental Illness and Other Characteristics, in L. Wynne et al. (Eds.), *The Nature of Schizophrenia: New Approaches to Research and Treatment* (pp. 25–37), New York: John Wiley & Sons.

16 Wender et al. (1974), Crossfostering: A Research Strategy for Clarifying the Role of Genetic and Experiential Factors in the Etiology of Schizophrenia, *Archives of General Psychiatry, 30,* 121–128. https://doi.org/10.1001/archpsyc .1974.01760070097016

17 Critical analyses of the Danish-American Crossfostering Study can be found in Boyle, M. (2002), *Schizophrenia: A Scientific Delusion?* (2nd ed.), Hove, UK: Routledge, pp. 192–194; Joseph, 2004, 2006; Lewontin, R. C., Rose, S., & Kamin, L. J. (1984), *Not in Our Genes: Biology, Ideology, and Human Nature,* New York: Pantheon, pp. 226–227.

18 Kety et al. (1968), The Types and Prevalence of Mental Illness in the Biological and Adoptive Families of Adopted Schizophrenics, in D. Rosenthal & S. Kety (Eds.), *The Transmission of Schizophrenia* (pp. 345–362), New York: Pergamon Press.

19 There were actually 34 index adoptees. One consisted of the members of an MZ twin pair adopted by the same parents, who were counted as one adoptee by the researchers.

20 Kety et al. 1968, p. 361.

21 Kety et al. (1975), Mental Illness in the Biological and Adoptive Families of Adopted Individuals who Have Become Schizophrenic: A Preliminary Report Based on Psychiatric Interviews, in R. Fieve et al. (Eds.), *Genetic Research in Psychiatry* (pp. 147–165), Baltimore: The Johns Hopkins Press.

22 One control adoptee was added to the 1975 study, because the researchers decided to count both control adoptees matched to the index adoptee MZ twin pair. This index twin pair was still counted as one index adoptee in the 1975 study.

23 Kety et al., 1975, p. 163.

24 Kety et al. (1978), Genetic Relationships within the Schizophrenia Spectrum: Evidence from Adoption Studies, in R. Spitzer & D. Klein (Eds.), *Critical Issues in Psychiatric Diagnosis* (pp. 213–223), New York: Raven Press; Kety et al. (1994), Mental Illness in the Biological and Adoptive Relatives of Schizophrenic Adoptees: Replication of the Copenhagen Study to the Rest of Denmark, *Archives of General Psychiatry, 51,* 442–455. https://doi.org/10.1001/archpsyc .1994.03950060006001

25 Kety et al., 1994, p. 442.

26 Rosenthal et al. (1968), Schizophrenics' Offspring Reared in Adoptive Homes, in D. Rosenthal & S. Kety (Eds.), *The Transmission of Schizophrenia* (pp. 377–391), New York: Pergamon Press; Rosenthal et al. (1971), The Adopted-Away Offspring of Schizophrenics, *American Journal of Psychiatry, 128,* p. 307. https://doi.org/10.1176/ajp.128.3.307.

27 Rosenthal et al., 1968, pp. 378, 380.

28 Rosenthal et al., 1971, p. 308.

29 Rosenthal et al., 1968, p. 386.

30 Rosenthal et al., 1971, p. 309.

31 Rosenthal et al., 1971, p. 309.

32 Rosenthal et al., 1971, p. 307.

33 Haier, R. J., Rosenthal, D., & Wender, P. H. (1978), MMPI Assessment of Psychopathology in the Adopted-Away Offspring of Schizophrenics, *Archives of General Psychiatry, 35,* 171–175, p. 174.

34 Tienari et al. (1987), Genetic and Psychosocial Factors in Schizophrenia: The Finnish Adoptive Family Study, *Schizophrenia Bulletin, 13,* 477–484. https:// doi.org/10.1093/schbul/13.3.477; Tienari et al. (2003), Genetic Boundaries of the Schizophrenia Spectrum: Evidence from the Finnish Adoptive Family Study, *American Journal of Psychiatry, 160,* 1587–1594. https://doi.org/10.1176/appi .ajp.160.9.1587

35 Based on figures from Tienari et al., 2003. In this 2003 publication (p. 1590), Tienari diagnosed DSM-III-R schizophrenia in 7 out of 137 index adoptees whose biological mothers were also diagnosed with DSM-III-R schizophrenia (5.1%). DSM-III-R schizophrenia was diagnosed in 3 of the 192 control adoptees (1.6%). Using Fisher's Exact Test, one-tailed, the probability value for this difference = .065, which is not statistically significant at the conventional .05 level of significance.

36 Tienari et al. (2004), Genotype-Environment Interaction in Schizophrenia-Spectrum Disorders, *British Journal of Psychiatry, 184,* 216–222, p. 216. https://doi.org/10.1192/bjp.184.3.216

37 Tienari et al. (1987), The Finnish Adoptive Family Study of Schizophrenia: Possible Joint Effects of Genetic Vulnerability and Family Interaction, in K. Halweg & M. Goldstein (Eds.), *Understanding Major Mental Disorder: The Contribution of Family Interaction Research* (pp. 33–54), New York: Family Process Press, pp. 44–45.

38 Tienari et al., 1987, Genetic and Psychosocial Factors in Schizophrenia, p. 478.

39 Documentation of problem areas 2–4 can be found in Joseph, 2004, pp. 261–271, and in the references therein.

40 For critical analyses of Tienari's study, see Boyle, M., 2002, pp. 194–199; Jackson, G. E. (2003), Rethinking the Finnish Adoption Studies of Schizophrenia: A Challenge to Genetic Determinism, *Journal of Critical Psychology, Counselling and Psychotherapy, 3,* 129–138; Joseph, 2004, Chapter 7, pp. 261–271.

41 Lichtenstein et al. (2009), Common Genetic Determinants of Schizophrenia and Bipolar Disorder in Swedish Families: A Population-Based Study, *Lancet, 373,* 234–239. https://doi.org/10.1016/S0140-6736(09)60072-6

42 Hansen, B. S. (1996), Something Rotten in the State of Denmark: Eugenics and the Ascent of the Welfare State, in G. Broberg & N. Roll-Hansen (Eds.), *Eugenics and the Welfare State: Sterilization Policy in Denmark, Sweden, Norway, and Finland* (pp. 9–76), East Lansing, MI: Michigan State University Press; Kemp, T. (1957), Genetic-Hygienic Experiences in Denmark in Recent Years, *Eugenics Review, 49,* 11–18. https://www.ncbi.nlm.nih.gov/labs/pmc/articles/PMC2973766/pdf/eugenrev00037-0018.pdf

43 Hansen, 1996.

44 Mother's Aid Organization for Copenhagen, Copenhagen County and Frederiksborg County, Annual Report for 1946–47. Quoted in Mednick, S. A., & Hutchings, B. (1977), Some Considerations in the Interpretation of the Danish Adoption Studies in Relation to Asocial Behavior, in S. Mednick & K. Christiansen (Eds.), *Biosocial Bases of Criminal Behavior* (pp. 159–164). New York: Gardner Press, p. 163.

45 Häfner, H., & der Heiden, W. (1986), The Contribution of European Case Registers to Research on Schizophrenia, *Schizophrenia Bulletin, 12,* 26–51. https://doi.org/10.1093/schbul/12.1.26

46 Kemp, 1957.

47 Mednick, S. A. (1996), General Discussion III, in G. Bock & J. Goode (Eds.), *Genetics of Criminal and Antisocial Behavior* (pp. 129–137), New York: John Wiley and Sons, p. 134.

48 Olson, C. P. (Ed.) (1920), *Oregon Laws: Showing All the Laws of a General Nature in Force in the State of Oregon* (Vol. 2), San Francisco: The Bancroft-Whitney Company. See also Joseph, 2004, pp. 204–212.

49 Olson, 1920, p. 3176.

50 Anonymous (1925), Galton Society, *Eugenical News, 10,* 69–71, p. 71.

51 Hemminki et al. (1997), Sterilization in Finland: From Eugenics to Contraception, *Social Science and Medicine, 45,* 1875–1884. https://doi.org/10.1016/s0277-9536(97)00126-3; Hietala, M. (1996), From Race Hygiene to

Sterilization: The Eugenics Movement in Finland, in G. Broberg & N. Roll-Hansen (Eds.), *Eugenics and the Welfare State* (pp. 195–258), East Lansing, MI: Michigan State University Press.

52 Broberg, G., & Tydén, M. (1996), Eugenics in Sweden: Efficient Care, in G. Broberg & N. Roll-Hansen (Eds.), *Eugenics and the Welfare State* (pp. 77–149), East Lansing, MI: Michigan State University Press.

53 Open Science Collaboration (2015), Psychology: Estimating the Reproducibility of Psychological Science, *Science, 349* (6251), aac4716-1- aac47168. https://doi .org/10.1126/science.aac4716

54 Open Science Collaboration, 2015, p. aac4716-1.

55 Critical analyses of the Danish-American schizophrenia adoption studies include Benjamin, L. S. (1976), A Reconsideration of the Kety and Associates Study of Genetic Factors in the Transmission of Schizophrenia, *American Journal of Psychiatry, 133,* 1129–1133. https://doi.org/10.1176/ajp.133.10.1129; Boyle, 2002; Cassou et al., 1980; Joseph, 2004, 2006; Joseph, 2013; Lewontin et al., 1984, Chapter 8; Lidz, T. (1976), Commentary on a Critical Review of Recent Adoption, Twin, and Family Studies of Schizophrenia: Behavioral Genetics Perspectives, *Schizophrenia Bulletin, 2,* 402–412. https://doi.org/10.1093/schbul /2.3.402; Lidz, T., & Blatt, S. (1983), Critique of the Danish-American Studies of the Biological and Adoptive Relatives of Adoptees who Became Schizophrenic, *American Journal of Psychiatry, 140,* 426–435. https://doi.org/10.1176/ajp.140 .4.426; Lidz, T., Blatt, S., & Cook, B. (1981), Critique of the Danish-American Studies of the Adopted-Away Offspring of Schizophrenic Parents, *American Journal of Psychiatry, 138,* 1063–1068. https://doi.org/10.1176/ajp.138.8.1063; Pam, A. (1995), Biological Psychiatry: Science or Pseudoscience?, in C. Ross & A. Pam (Eds.), *Pseudoscience in Biological Psychiatry: Blaming the Body* (pp. 7–84), New York: John Wiley & Sons.

56 Examples of "independent" analyses of the Danish-American studies based on DSM-III diagnostic criteria include Lowing, P. A., Mirsky, A. F., & Pereira, R. (1983), The Inheritance of Schizophrenia Spectrum Disorders: A Reanalysis of the Danish Adoptee Study Data, *American Journal of Psychiatry, 140,* 1167– 117. https://doi.org/10.1176/ajp.140.9.1167; Kendler, K. S., & Gruenberg, A. M. (1984), An Independent Analysis of the Danish Adoption Study of Schizophrenia, *Archives of General Psychiatry, 41,* 555–564. https://doi.org /10.1001/archpsyc.1984.01790170029004; Kendler, K. S., Gruenberg, A. M., & Kinney, D. K. (1994), Independent Diagnoses of Adoptees and Relatives as Defined by DSM-III in the Provincial and National Samples of the Danish Adoption Study of Schizophrenia, *Archives of General Psychiatry, 51,* 456–468. https://doi.org/10.1001/archpsyc.1994.03950060020002

57 Kirk, S. A., Gomory, T., & Cohen, D. (2013), *Mad Science: Psychiatric Coercion, Diagnosis, and Drugs,* New Brunswick, NJ: Transaction.

58 In a 1975 publication, Rosenthal described how he and his colleagues searched through the "*APA Diagnostic and Statistical Manual,* second edition" (DSM-II) to select the spectrum disorders they used in their studies. See Rosenthal, D. (1975), The Spectrum Concept in Schizophrenic and Manic-Depressive Disorders, in D. Freedman (Ed.), *Biology of the Major Psychoses* (pp. 19–25), New York: Raven Press, pp. 19–20. In February of 1967, a pre-publication draft of the DSM-II was distributed to psychiatrists. See American Psychiatric Association (1968), *Diagnostic and Statistical Manual of Mental Disorders* (2nd ed. [DSM-II]), Washington, DC: American Psychiatric Association, p. ix.

59 Kety et al., 1968, pp. 351–352.

60 Kety, S. S. (1974), From Rationalization to Reason, *American Journal of Psychiatry, 131,* 957–963, p. 960. https://doi.org/10.1176/ajp.131.9.957

61 Kety, S. S. (1987), The Significance of Genetic Factors in the Etiology of Schizophrenia: Results from the National Study of Adoptees in Denmark, *Journal of Psychiatric Research, 21,* 423–429, p. 424. https://doi.org/10.1016 /0022-3956(87)90089-6

62 Flint, J., Greenspan, R. J., & Kendler, K. S. (2020), *How Genes Influence Behavior* (2nd ed.), Oxford, UK: Oxford University Press, pp. 9–10.

63 Jauhar, S., Johnstone, M., & McKenna, P. J. (2022), Schizophrenia, *Lancet, 399,* 473–486, p. 474. https://doi.org/10.1016/S0140-6736(21)01730-X

64 Kety et al., 1968, p. 352

65 Kety et al. (1976), Studies Based on a Total Sample of Adopted Individuals and their Relatives: Why They Were Necessary, What They Demonstrated and Failed to Demonstrate, *Schizophrenia Bulletin, 2,* 413–428, p. 420. https://doi .org/10.1093/schbul/2.3.413

66 Kety, S. S. (1983), Mental Illness in the Biological and Adoptive Relatives of Schizophrenia Adoptees: Findings Relevant to Genetic and Environmental Factors in Etiology, *American Journal of Psychiatry, 140,* 720–727, p. 724. https://doi.org/10.1176/ajp.140.6.720

67 Kety, S. S. (1983), Dr. Kety Responds [Letter to the Editor], *American Journal of Psychiatry, 140,* 964, p. 964. https://doi.org/10.1176/ajp.140.7.964

68 Rosenthal, 1975, The Spectrum Concept, p. 19.

69 Rosenthal, D. (1979), Genetic Factors in Behavioural Disorders, in M. Roth & V. Cowie (Eds.), *Psychiatry, Genetics and Pathography: A Tribute to Eliot Slater* (pp. 22–33), London: Oxford University Press, p. 23.

70 The mid-20th-century chronic schizophrenia rate in the Danish population has been given as 0.69 percent. See Slater, E., & Cowie, V. (1971), *The Genetics of Mental Disorders,* London: Oxford University Press, p. 13. For more details, see Joseph, 2006, Chapter 3.

71 Rosenthal, D. (1972), Three Adoption Studies of Heredity in the Schizophrenic Disorders, *International Journal of Mental Health, 1,* 63–75, p. 65. https://doi .org/10.1080/00207411.1972.11448565

72 Rosenthal, D. (1971), A Program of Research on Heredity in Schizophrenia, *Behavioral Science, 16,* 191–201. https://doi.org/10.1002/bs.3830160302, p. 194.

73 In 1994, Kety and colleagues wrote, "Prospective [Danish] adoptive parents were screened for mental health and economic stability by the courts and a history or current indication of mental illness in either biological parent would favor a legal abortion or a decision not to place the child for adoption." Kety et al., 1994, p. 452.

74 Joseph, 2006.

75 Joseph, 2006, Chapter 3. See also Joseph, 2004, Chapter 7.

76 Rosenthal, 1972, Three Adoption Studies, pp. 68–69.

77 Ingraham, L. J., & Kety, S. S. (1988), Schizophrenia Spectrum Disorders, in M. Tsuang & J. Simpson (Eds.), *Handbook of Schizophrenia, Vol. 3: Nosology, Epidemiology and Genetics* (pp. 117–137), New York: Elsevier Science Publishers, pp. 121–123.

78 Head et al. (2015), The Extent and Consequences of P-Hacking in Science, *PLoS Biology, 13(3):* e1002106. https://doi.org/10.1371/journal.pbio.1002106

79 American Psychiatric Association, 1968, p. 44.

80 Szasz, T. S. (1976), *Schizophrenia: The Sacred Symbol of Psychiatry,* New York: Basic Books, p. xiv.

81 Kety et al., 1975, p. 154.

82 Rosenthal et al., 1968, p. 387. This index adoptee's complete "schizophrenia spectrum diagnosis" was listed as "border-line schizophrenia or pervert."

83 Rosenthal et al. (1975), Assessing Degree of Psychopathology from Diagnostic Statements, *Canadian Psychiatric Association Journal, 20,* 35–45. https://doi.org/10.1177/070674377502000107, p. 40; Wender et al., 1974, p. 124, Table 2.

84 Kety et al., 1968, p. 252, Table 3.

85 American Psychiatric Association, 1968, pp. 33–35.

86 Kety et al., 1968, p. 353.

87 Kety, 1959, p. 1594.

88 Rosenthal, D. (1967), An Historical and Methodological Review of Genetic Studies of Schizophrenia, in J. Romano (Ed.), *The Origins of Schizophrenia: Proceedings of the First Rochester International Conference on Schizophrenia, March 29–31, 1967* (pp. 15–26), New York: Excerpta Medica Foundation, p. 25.

89 Kety et al., 1968, p. 346.

90 Kety et al., 1968, p. 358, Table 5.

91 Kety et al., 1968, p. 353.

92 Lidz & Blatt, 1983, pp. 426–427.

93 Lidz, T., Fleck, S., & Cornelison, A. R. (1965), *Schizophrenia and the Family,* New York: International Universities Press.

94 Lidz, T. (1967), The Family, Personality Development, and Schizophrenia, in J. Romano (Ed.), *The Origins of Schizophrenia: Proceedings of the First Rochester International Conference on Schizophrenia, March 29–31, 1967* (pp. 131–138), New York: Excerpta Medica Foundation. There is a photograph of Lidz and other Rochester conference attendees, including David Rosenthal, on page viii of this book.

95 Andreasen, N. C. (1984), *The Broken Brain: The Biological Revolution in Psychiatry,* New York: Harper & Row, pp. 29–30.

96 Lidz & Blatt, 1983, p. 426.

97 Kety, 1983, Mental Illness in the Biological and Adoptive Relatives of Schizophrenia Adoptees. p. 721.

98 Kety, 1983, Dr. Kety Responds, p. 964.

99 Kety, 1974, p. 961.

100 Munafò et al. (2017), A Manifesto for Reproducible Science, *Nature Human Behaviour, 1,* 0021, p. 2. https://doi.org/10.1038/s41562-016-0021

101 Kendler & Gruenberg, 1984, p. 556.

102 Lewontin et al., 1984, p. 224.

103 Jacobs, D. (1994), Environmental Failure—Oppression Is the Only Cause of Psychopathology, *Journal of Mind and Behavior, 15,* 1–18, p. 8.

104 Paikin et al. (1974), Characteristics of People Who Refused to Participate in a Social and Psychopathological Study, in S. Mednick et al. (Eds.), *Genetics, Environment and Psychopathology* (pp. 293–322), New York: American Elsevier, pp. 308–310.

105 Kety et al., 1968, p. 354.

106 For example, Kety, Rosenthal, and Wender wrote that chronic schizophrenia "is the only syndrome which merits the designation of schizophrenia in Denmark"; see Kety et al., 1978, Genetic Relationships Within the Schizophrenia Spectrum, p. 214.

107 Rosenthal, 1972, pp. 73–74.

108 Kety et al., 1975, p. 154.

109 Kety et al., 1975, p. 158.

110 The original B1 diagnosis for the biological father of control adoptee C9 is found in Kety et al., 1968, p. 355. In Kety et al., 1975, p. 160, he was listed as a biological father, along with his 1968 B1 diagnosis and a notation that he had subsequently died.

111 B1 rates of 5/173 index versus 1/174 control produce a probability value of .11 (Fisher's Exact Test, one-tailed), which is not statistically significant at the conventional .05 level of statistical significance used by the Danish-American researchers.

112 Ingraham & Kety, 1988, p. 122, Table 1.

113 Kety et al., 1975, p. 154.

114 Benjamin, 1976, p. 1130.

115 Kety et al., 1975, p. 163, Table 6.

116 Boyle, 2002, pp. 186–187. Family diagnostic counts are based on data in Kety et al., 1975, pp. 158–161 (Tables 4a and 4b). There are 8 index biological families out of 33 with at least one B1, B2, or B3 diagnosis, versus 3 control biological families out of 34 with at least one B1, B2, or B3 diagnosis (see pp. 158–161). This comparison is not statistically significant at the conventional .05 level (index families 8/33 vs. control families 3/34, Fisher's Exact Test, one-tailed, p = .084). For the B and D diagnoses combined, the comparison remains statistically non-significant (index families 11/33 vs. control families 5/34, Fisher's Exact Test, one-tailed, p = .066).

117 Boyle, 2002, p. 186.

118 Kety et al., 1975, p. 156.

119 Kety et al., 1975, p. 156.

120 Kety et al., 1975, p. 156.

121 Kety et al., 1975, p. 156.

122 Source: Based on totals provided in Kety et al., 1975, p. 162.

123 Joseph, 2004; Lidz & Blatt, 1983. Kety and colleagues continued to count Category C "schizoid or inadequate personality" as a schizophrenia spectrum disorder in the 1975 Kety-led study. In Table 3 of the Kety et al. 1975 publication (p. 154), Category C was located under the "Schizophrenia spectrum" heading, and the 26 Category C index and control biological relative diagnoses were included among the 56 index and control biological relative diagnoses falling into the clearly marked "Total in schizophrenia spectrum" category. On page 155 they wrote, "We are not prepared to dismiss the possibility that there is a schizoid or inadequate personality which is genetically related to schizophrenia." In a different 1975 publication (found in the same edited book), Rosenthal defended the retention of Category C in the spectrum. See Rosenthal, D. (1975), Discussion: The Concept of Schizophrenic Disorders, in R. Fieve et al. (Eds.), *Genetic Research in Psychiatry* (pp. 199–208), Baltimore: The Johns Hopkins Press.

124 Kety et al., 1976, p. 418, Table 2a. Schizophrenia spectrum disorders, including the "Category C" schizoid/inadequate diagnosis, as were listed in this publication's Table 2a as 18/63 index, versus 11/64 control, with the probability value given as .094.

125 Based on totals provided in Kety et al. (1976), Studies Based on a Total Sample of Adopted Individuals and their Relatives: Why They Were Necessary, What They Demonstrated and Failed to Demonstrate, *Schizophrenia Bulletin, 2*, 413–428, p. 418. https://doi.org/10.1093/schbul/2.3.413.

126 Kety, S. S., Rosenthal, D., & Wender, P. H. (1978), Genetic Relationships Within the Schizophrenia Spectrum: Evidence from Adoption Studies, in R. Spitzer & D. Klein (Eds.), *Critical Issues in Psychiatric Diagnosis* (pp. 213–223), New York: Raven Press, p. 217.

127 Kety, S. S. (1985), The Adoption Strategy for Examining Genetic and Environmental Factors in Mental Disorder, in T. Sakai & T. Tsuboi (Eds.), *Genetic Aspects of Human Behavior* (pp. 157–164). New York: Igaku-Shoin, p. 160.

128 Ingraham, L. J., & Kety, S. S. (1988), Schizophrenia Spectrum Disorders, in M. Tsuang & J. Simpson (Eds.), *Handbook of Schizophrenia, Vol. 3: Nosology, Epidemiology and Genetics* (pp. 117–137), New York: Elsevier Science Publishers, p. 122.

129 Kety, S., & Ingraham, L. J. (1992), Genetic Transmission and Improved Diagnosis of Schizophrenia from Pedigrees of Adoptees, *Journal of Psychiatric Research, 26,* 247–255. https://doi.org/10.1016/0022-3956(92)90031-i

130 Kety et al., 1994, p. 448.

131 Jekel et al. (2007), *Epidemiology, Biostatistics, and Preventive Medicine* (3rd ed.), Philadelphia: Saunders-Elsevier, p. 206.

132 Flint, Greenspan, & Kendler, 2020, p. 295.

133 In the subsequent Kety-led 1994 final Provincial Study publication (pp. 448–450, Figures 1–3), by my count 6 of the 48 index biological paternal half-siblings were diagnosed with a schizophrenia spectrum disorder, versus 1 of the 28 control biological paternal half-siblings. The difference is not statistically significant (p = .19, Fisher's Exact Test, one-tailed), even though on page 453 Kety and colleagues stated, without supplying any numbers, that the Provincial Study index-control difference was statistically significant: "In both the Copenhagen and the Provincial Samples, the prevalence of chronic or latent schizophrenia in the paternal biological half-siblings was at least as high as in the maternal half-siblings, and significantly higher than in their controls." In fact, the biological paternal half-sibling schizophrenia spectrum disorder comparison was statistically non-significant in *both* samples.

134 Kety et al., 1978, Genetic Relationships within the Schizophrenia Spectrum, p. 217.

135 Kety, 1983, Mental Illness in the Biological and Adoptive Relatives of Schizophrenia Adoptees, p. 723.

136 Kety, 1983, Mental Illness in the Biological and Adoptive Relatives of Schizophrenia Adoptees, p. 723.

137 Kety, 1985, p. 160.

138 Ingraham & Kety, 1988, p. 122.

139 Kety & Ingraham, 1992, p. 248.

140 Kety et al., 1994, p. 450.

141 Kety, S. S. (1983), Observations on Genetic and Environmental Influences in the Etiology of Mental Disorder from Studies on Adoptees and their Relatives, in S. Kety et al. (Eds.), *Genetics of Neurological and Psychiatric Disorders* (pp. 105–114), New York: Raven Press, p. 109.

142 Kety et al., 1994, p. 446.

143 Kety et al., 1975, pp. 155–156.

144 Kendler, Gruenberg, & Kinney, 1994, p. 459; Kety et al., 1994, p. 451.

145 Kendler, Gruenberg, & Kinney, 1994, p. 457.

146 Kendler, Gruenberg, & Kinney, 1994, p. 467.

147 Kety et al., 1994, p. 454.

148 Kendler, K. S., & Diehl, S. R. (1993), The Genetics of Schizophrenia: A Current, Genetic-Epidemiologic Perspective, *Schizophrenia Bulletin, 19,* 261–285, p. 265. https://doi.org/10.1093/schbul/19.2.261

149 Kendler, Gruenberg, & Kinney, 1994, p. 459, Table 2.

150 Kendler, Gruenberg, & Kinney, 1994, p. 460, Table 3.

151 Joseph, 2004, p. 243; Kety et al., 1994, p. 448.

152 Kety et al., 1994, p. 447, Table 3. See also Joseph, 2004, 2006.

153 The family of chronic schizophrenia index adoptee "069." See Kety et al., 1994, p. 448, Figure 1.

154 Rosenthal et al., 1968, p. 387.

155 Rosenthal et al., 1968, p. 388.
156 Rosenthal et al., 1968, pp. 390–391.
157 Rosenthal et al., 1968, p. 389.
158 Rosenthal et al., 1968, p. 391.
159 Rosenthal, D. (1971), *Genetics of Psychopathology*, New York: McGraw-Hill, p. 81.
160 Ritchie, S. (2020), *Science Fictions: How Fraud, Bias, Negligence, and Hype Undermine the Search for Truth*, Henry Holt and Co.
161 See Rosenthal et al., 1971, p. 309.
162 Rosenthal, 1971, p. 124.
163 Rosenthal et al., 1971. For more on this point, see Joseph 2004; Lidz et al., 1981.
164 Rosenthal et al., 1971, p. 309.
165 Kety et al., 1976, p. 417.
166 Rosenthal et al., 1971, p. 309.
167 Rosenthal et al., 1968, p. 382.
168 Pam, 1995, p. 31.
169 Lidz et al., 1981, p. 1064.
170 Haier et al., 1978, p. 174. The Haier et al. 1978 investigator-defined schizophrenia spectrum consisted of chronic schizophrenia, borderline schizophrenia, and "schizophrenic personality." The results, as seen in Table 3 of this publication, counted 21/60 (35%) of the index adoptees with a spectrum disorder diagnosis, versus 16/62 (26%) of the control adoptees. The index-control difference is not statistically significant (p = .18, Fisher's Exact Test, one-tailed).
171 Haier et al., 1978, p. 171.
172 Lewontin et al., 1984, p. 226.
173 John, L. K., Loewenstein, G., & Prelec, D. (2012), Measuring the Prevalence of Questionable Research Practices with Incentives for Truth Telling, *Psychological Science, 23,* 524–532. https://doi.org/10.1177/0956797611430953
174 Based on QRPs described in John et al., 2012.
175 Leo, J., & Joseph, J. (2002), Schizophrenia: Medical Students Are Taught It's All in the Genes, But Are They Hearing the Whole Story?, *Ethical Human Sciences and Services, 4,* 17–30.
176 Kaplan, H. I., & Sadock, B. J. (1996), *Concise Textbook of Clinical Psychiatry* (1st ed.), Baltimore: Williams & Wilkins, p. 127.
177 Choudary, P. V., & Knowles, J. A. (2008), Genetics, in R. Hales et al. (Eds.), *The American Psychiatric Publishing Textbook of Psychiatry* (5th ed.; pp. 191–243), Washington DC: American Psychiatric Publications, p. 210; Knowles, J. A. (2003), Genetics, in R. Hales et al. (Eds.), *The American Psychiatric Publishing Textbook of Clinical Psychiatry* (4th ed.; pp. 3–65), Washington DC: American Psychiatric Publications, p. 20.
178 Minzenberg et al. (2011), Schizophrenia, in R. E. Hales et al. (Eds.), *Essentials of Psychiatry* (3rd ed.; pp. 111–150), Washington, DC: American Psychiatric Publishing, p. 126.
179 Kendler, K. S. (1988), The Genetics of Schizophrenia: An Overview, in M. Tsuang & J. Simpson (Eds.), *Handbook of Schizophrenia, Vol. 3: Nosology, Epidemiology and Genetics* (pp. 437–462), New York: Elsevier Science Publishers, p. 447.
180 Kety et al., 1976, p. 420.
181 Kety et al. (1971), Mental Illness in the Biological and Adoptive Families of Adopted Schizophrenics, *American Journal of Psychiatry, 128,* 302–306, p. 302. https://doi.org/10.1176/ajp.128.3.302
182 Ridley, M. (2004), *The Agile Gene: How Nature Turns on Nurture* [Originally published as *Nature via Nurture*], New York: Perennial, pp. 105–106.

183 Egan, M. F., & Hyde, T. M. (2000), Schizophrenia: Neurobiology, in B. Sadock & V. Sadock (Eds.), *Kaplan & Sadock's Comprehensive Textbook of Psychiatry* (7th ed., Vol. 1; pp. 1129–1147), Philadelphia: Lippincott, Williams, & Wilkins, p. 1130; Sadock, B. J., & Sadock, V. A. (2008), *Concise Textbook of Clinical Psychiatry* (3rd ed.), Philadelphia: Lippincott, Williams & Wilkins, p. 158.

184 Gurling, H. M. D., & McQuillin, A. (2012), The Genetics of Schizophrenia, in J. I. Nurnberger & W. H. Berrettini (Eds.), *Principles of Psychiatric Genetics* (pp. 230–261), Cambridge, UK: Cambridge University Press, p. 237; Kennedy et al. (1989), Molecular Genetic Studies in Schizophrenia, *Schizophrenia Bulletin, 15,* 383–391, p. 383; Lyons et al., 1991, p. 125; Cardno, A. & McGuffin, P. (2003), Quantitative Genetics, in P. McGuffin et al. (Eds.), *Psychiatric Genetics and Genomics* (pp. 35–53), Oxford: Oxford University Press, p. 35; Maxmen, J. S., & Ward, N. G. (1995), *Essential Psychopathology and Its Treatment* (2nd ed., revised for DSM-IV), New York: W. W. Norton, pp. 70–71; McGuffin et al. (1994), *Seminars in Psychiatric Genetics*, London: Gaskell Press, p. 35; Owen, M. J., & O'Donovan, M. C. (2003), Schizophrenia and Genetics, in R. Plomin, J. DeFries, I. Craig, & P. McGuffin (Eds.), *Behavioral Genetics in the Postgenomic Era* (pp. 463–480), Washington, DC: American Psychological Association Press, p. 465; Owen, M. J., O'Donovan, M. C., & Gottesman, I. I. (2003), Schizophrenia, in P. McGuffin et al. (Eds.), *Psychiatric Genetics and Genomics* (pp. 247–266), Oxford: Oxford University Press, p. 249; Riley, B., Asherson, P., & McGuffin, P. (2003), Genetics and Schizophrenia, in S. Hirsch & D. Weinberger (Eds.), *Schizophrenia* (pp. 251–276), Malden, MA: Blackwell, p. 255; Sullivan, P. F. (2005), The Genetics of Schizophrenia, *PLOS Medicine, July, 2(7),* 0614–0618 (see Table 1 of this publication). https://doi.org/10.1371/journal.pmed.0020212; Tandon, R., Keshavan, M. S., & Nasrallah, H. A. (2008), Schizophrenia "Just the Facts": What We Know in 2008, 2, Epidemiology and Etiology, *Schizophrenia Research, 102,* 1–18, p. 5. https://doi.org/10.1016/j.schres.2008.04.011; Tsuang, M. T., & Vandermey, R. (1980), *Genes and the Mind: Inheritance of Mental Illness*, Oxford: Oxford University Press, p. 59.

185 DeLisi, L. E. (2017), *100 Questions & Answers About Schizophrenia: Painful Minds* (3rd ed.), Burlington, MA: Jones & Bartlett, p. 95.

186 DeLisi, L. E. (2022), Redefining Schizophrenia Through Genetics: A Commentary on 50 Years Searching for Biological Causes, *Schizophrenia Research, 242,* 22–24. https://doi.org/10.1016/j.schres.2021.11.017

187 Freedman, R. (2010), *The Madness Within Us: Schizophrenia as a Neuronal Process*, New York: Oxford University Press, p. 79.

188 Kety et al., 1971.

189 Kolker, 2020, *Hidden Valley Road: Inside the Mind of an American Family*. New York: Anchor, p. 116.

190 Kolker, 2020, p. 117.

191 Kolker, 2020, Chapter 9.

192 Lieberman, J., & Ogas, O. (2016, March 3), Genetics and Mental Illness—Let's Not Get Carried Away, *Wall Street Journal*. https://www.wsj.com/articles/genetics-and-mental-illnesslets-not-get-carried-away-1457048745. See also Joseph, J. (2016, March 21), Comments on Jeffrey Lieberman and Ogi Ogas' *Wall Street Journal* Article on the Genetics of Psychiatric Disorders, [Web log post, *Mad in America* "The Gene Illusion"]. https://www.madinamerica.com/2016/03/comments-on-jeffrey-lieberman-and-ogi-ogas-wall-street-journal-article-on-the-genetics-of-psychiatric-disorders/

193 Lieberman et al. (Eds.) (2020), *The American Psychiatric Publishing Textbook of Schizophrenia* (2nd ed.), Washington, DC: American Psychiatric Publishing.

194 Joseph, 2006, Chapter 7, pp., 125–127.

195 Lieberman, J., & Ogas, O. (2015), *Shrinks: The Untold Story of Psychiatry*, New York: Little Brown, p. 231.
196 Joseph, 2006, pp. 77–78.
197 For elaboration on these points, see Boyle, 2002; Joseph, 2004, 2006.
198 Rosenthal, D. (1974), The Concept of Subschizophrenic Disorders, in S. Mednick, et al. (Eds.), *Genetics, Environment, & Psychopathology* (pp. 167–176), New York: American Elsevier, p. 167. Rosenthal's use of the term "Pandora's box" in reference to creating the schizophrenia spectrum is taken directly from this publication.
199 Bentall, R. P. (2009), *Doctoring the Mind: Is Our Current Treatment of Mental Illness Really Any Good?*, New York: New York University Press, p. 124.
200 Gould, S. J. (1981), *The Mismeasure of Man*, New York: W. W. Norton, pp. 89, 102.

7 Schizophrenia and Genetics
Conclusions and Future Directions

A major theme of this book has been that schizophrenia genetic research must be evaluated in the larger context of the replication crisis in science. The QRP concept now provides a framework to help bring faulty research into the light. In previous chapters, I showed how schizophrenia genetic research has been characterized by QRPs such as p-hacking and HARKing, by a reliance on false or highly questionable assumptions in twin research and other areas, and by spurious or non-causative gene-associations. The QRP framework provides an increasingly accepted language describing how and where research goes wrong—at times terribly wrong.

I conclude that there exists no scientifically acceptable evidence that schizophrenia or psychosis have an underlying genetic basis, which has implications for most other areas of human behavior. Using behavioral genetic and psychiatric genetic terminology, over 100 years of research has failed to produce reliable evidence that schizophrenia/psychosis is heritable. If researchers of the future produce genetic findings based on sound pre-registered research and validated assumptions, and are able to eliminate or control for environmental confounds, such findings will be evaluated when they appear.

We saw in Chapter 1 that some have rejected the idea that schizophrenia is a valid medical disorder or "disease." Losing the genetic component will seriously undercut support for the disease model. Once the schizophrenia genetic domino falls, many other genetics of behavior dominoes may fall as well. The fields of psychiatry, psychiatric genetics, and behavioral genetics will see this as a threat to their existence; drug companies will worry about their profits; and establishment political parties begrudgingly will need to direct much more government funding toward improving people's lives. The rest of the world will be content to let the dominoes fall.

A future widespread recognition that "schizophrenia" is not genetic or "heritable," and that it is not a disease, will be a reason to celebrate. Society will then part ways with genetic diversions and inappropriate medical approaches, and will instead focus on environmental causes, non-medical interventions, and prevention. Because family, social, cultural, religious, educational, geographical, and political environments together play

DOI: 10.4324/9781003293279-7

a powerful role in shaping human behavior, attention will be focused away from people's brains and genes, and toward aspects of the environment that on the one hand help protect, nurture, and empower people, and on the other hand can psychologically harm people.

Chapter Summaries

Before looking at alternative understandings of the schizophrenia concept, in addition to non-medical prevention and intervention strategies, I will summarize the first six chapters of this book.

I introduced the schizophrenia genetics topic in *Chapter 1*, and listed the main research methods used to support the "high heritability" of schizophrenia and psychosis: family studies, twin studies, adoption studies, and molecular genetic studies. I then showed that the "genetics of schizophrenia" question has much larger implications relating to the nature-nurture debate, which was followed by a discussion of the history of the schizophrenia concept and the controversies surrounding it. I then introduced the field of psychiatric genetics, and examined problems with genetic explanations of schizophrenia. The chapter ended with a discussion of the ongoing replication crisis in the behavioral sciences and elsewhere, and its relevance to a proper understanding of the schizophrenia genetic research analyzed in subsequent chapters.

Chapter 2 began with a brief overview of schizophrenia molecular genetic research. I showed that the practice of estimating heritability is faulty, and that a heritability estimate does not tell us "how much" genes influence schizophrenia and other types of behavior. Schizophrenia heritability estimates, therefore, have little or no meaning. I then explored different eras of schizophrenia molecular genetic research, including the failed linkage and candidate gene eras, leading up to the current genome-wide association/ polygenic risk score era. Despite countless gene discovery claims in the media and in academic works since the 1970s, genes shown to cause schizophrenia and psychosis have not been found. The failure to discover causative genes creates an additional reason to re-examine the body of family, twin, and adoption research that had supposedly established the "high heritability of schizophrenia." *The belief that these studies established schizophrenia as a genetically based disease is the fundamental error of schizophrenia genefinding strategies.*

Chapter 3 looked only briefly at schizophrenia family studies due to the consensus view that a behavior or condition "running in the family" cannot be interpreted on genetic grounds. This is also seen in Irving Gottesman's famous 1991 schizophrenia risk percentage figure, which also cannot be interpreted on genetic grounds. I explored the origins of the psychiatric genetics field in Germany, and how Ernst Rüdin, the founding leader of this field, was involved in some of the crimes committed by the National Socialist regime. I looked at the large-sample schizophrenia family study by psychiatric geneticist Franz Kallmann, and described the findings of the more methodologically sound modern family studies. Finally, I reviewed Robert Kolker's 2020 *Hidden Valley Road*, a book about a family in which six children grew up to experience psychosis.

Chapter 4 began with a description of the classical twin method comparison of reared-together MZ and same-sex DZ twin pairs, and emphasized the importance of the twin method's MZ-DZ "equal environment assumption" (EEA). Although there is widespread agreement that MZ pairs grow up experiencing much more similar environments than DZs, twin researchers and their supporters have used various arguments in attempts to sidestep the twin method's unequal environments problem. I showed that none of these arguments supports the validity of the EEA. After briefly reviewing a widely cited twin study meta-analysis, I examined four major problems with the "EEA-test" literature. I ended the chapter by concluding that the results of behavioral studies using the twin method cannot be interpreted genetically—a conclusion that has major implications for schizophrenia twin research.

The main argument in *Chapter 5* was built on the conclusions I reached in the previous chapter. Because the EEA is false, schizophrenia twin studies cannot be interpreted genetically. The pooled pairwise MZ concordance rate is only around 24 percent in the more methodologically sound studies, compared with the pooled 4 percent DZ rate. The difference cannot be interpreted on genetic grounds, and these results show that when one MZ twin is diagnosed with schizophrenia, about 75 percent of the time their genetically identical MZ co-twin is not so diagnosed. I performed a critical review of a widely cited schizophrenia twin study meta-analysis, as well as the most recently published schizophrenia twin study. I then described the tragic story of the "Genain Quadruplets," and showed how researchers committed to genetic theories can overlook the potentially crazy-making impact of severe abuse experienced by siblings trapped in an inescapable situation. The misreporting of schizophrenia twin research in Siddhartha Mukherjee's *The Gene: An Intimate History* provides an example of problems in secondary-source reporting of schizophrenia genetic research. I described the offspring of discordant MZ pairs design, as well as anecdotal single-case reports of supposedly reared-apart MZ pairs concordant for schizophrenia. The limitations of both methods were noted. Overall, twin research has failed to provide scientifically acceptable evidence that genes play a role in causing schizophrenia and psychosis.

Chapter 6 explored schizophrenia adoption research, and focused on the two most frequently cited studies: the Kety-led and Rosenthal-led Danish-American investigations. I outlined several potentially confounding aspects of psychiatric adoption research, including selective placement, late separation, late placement, range restriction and the screening of adoptive families, and shared pre-natal environment. I showed that the Danish-American researchers used multiple QRPs across multiple studies to achieve statistically significant results in the genetic direction. Finally, I documented misleading accounts of these studies in many influential secondary-source publications. The Danish-American schizophrenia adoption studies are perhaps the longest running example of p-hacked research ever seen in the behavioral sciences, and these studies should be retracted. In addition, for reasons discussed in the chapter, the results of the remaining schizophrenia adoption studies cannot be interpreted genetically.

Psychiatric Genetics: A Future "Null Field"?

We saw in Chapter 2 that a *null field* is an area of scientific research "with absolutely no yield of true scientific information ... .The extent that observed findings deviate from what is expected by chance alone would be simply a pure measure of the prevailing bias."[1] In Chapter 2 I explored the idea that psychiatric genetics is or might one day become a null field, meaning that due to the field's "prevailing biases," the final verdict would be that it provided no yield of true scientific information about genetic influences on the psychiatric conditions it has studied in its 100+ years of existence.

Psychiatric genetics will become a recognized null field if one or both of the following occur. (1) The field decides to throw in the towel and shut down after decades of failed attempts to discover causative genes, and after funding sources dry up. (2) Other areas of science conclude that psychiatric genetics is a null field after determining that its supposed findings represented nothing more than a "pure measure of the prevailing bias" in that field.

We saw in Chapter 3 that psychiatric genetic research began with Ernst Rüdin's genetically misinterpreted 1916 schizophrenia family study, which was followed by a 1920s manic-depression family study where Rüdin, the "father of psychiatric genetics," chose to suppress his findings because they failed to support psychiatric genetic and eugenic positions. It hasn't been necessary to suppress the results of psychiatric genetic research since that time, as the corrupted process I described in Chapter 1 has allowed genetic interpretations of massively flawed studies based on false or questionable assumptions to be incorporated into the teachings of mainstream psychiatry, psychology, and other fields—with the blessing, assistance, and financial support of the drug industry.

While providing no findings beneficial to the human condition, in various ways psychiatric genetics has harmed people not only because of its eugenic ("racial hygiene") history and origins, but because it has helped society and science divert attention from non-genetic causes of human suffering and dysfunction. Modern psychiatric geneticists, as did their predecessors in Rüdin's era, believe that although environmental influences play some role in causing psychiatric conditions, genetic influences predominate. The main difference between psychiatric genetics then and now is that its modern supporters arrive at a different set of conclusions and policy recommendations than did their predecessors in Rüdin's time. The common thread is that psychiatric genetic conclusions, policy recommendations, and practices have always been based on bad science.

The following passage is taken from Richard Bentall's 2009 book *Doctoring the Mind: Is Our Current Treatment of Mental Illness Really Any Good?* I have quoted it before, but it's worth repeating here because it is as relevant now as when it was written:

> No patient, not a single one, has ever benefited from genetic research into mental illness, although many have been indirectly harmed by it (because it has discouraged the development of adequate services for patients and, during one shameful period, was used to justify their slaughter). No effective treatments have so far been devised on the basis of genetic information and, given what we now know, it seems very unlikely that further research into the genetics of psychosis will lead to important therapeutic advances in the future.[2]

A mainstream admission of failure is found in a 2017 statement by Thomas Insel, former head of the NIMH:

> I spent 13 years at N.I.M.H. really pushing on the neuroscience and genetics of mental disorders, and when I look back on that, I realize that while I think I succeeded at getting lots of really cool papers published by cool scientists at fairly large costs—I think $20 billion—I don't think we moved the needle in reducing suicide, reducing hospitalizations, improving recovery for the tens of millions of people who have mental illness.[3]

The take-home point: $20 billion dollars wasted. As sociologist Andrew Scull wrote in the context of psychiatric research, "Genetics and neuroscience have flourished within the confines of universities, but their therapeutic payoff has been minimal or nonexistent."[4] The most charitable description of the psychiatric genetics field is that it has produced minimal or nonexistent payoffs after over a century of trying.

Given this reality, people and groups that have questioned genetic claims and the schizophrenia concept itself, and have promoted non-medical intervention and prevention approaches, deserve a much wider hearing. It is to these areas that I now turn.

Alternative Understandings of "Schizophrenia" and Psychosis

There is a wide range of opinions about the causes of schizophrenia and psychosis. On one side is the genetic determinist view that behaviors associated with schizophrenia are symptoms of a disease process in the brain, and that genes are the main cause of this disease process. A role for environmental factors or triggers is acknowledged but greatly deemphasized. Many psychiatrists and schizophrenia genetic researchers hold this view.

In contrast, the environmentalist position I and others support makes the case that there is little evidence supporting the concept of "schizophrenia" or the brain disease model, and that the genetic evidence is weak or nonexistent. People's experiences are much better characterized by the term *psychosis*. The environmentalist position sees genetic research as a huge waste of money and resources, and as a distraction from the need to focus on identified environmental influences. Non-medical interventions are promoted to help people deal with or overcome distressing feelings, thoughts, and behaviors. The main way to reduce psychological distress and dysfunction (which psychiatry calls "psychopathology") is to improve environmental conditions and promote political change. People have the right to take prescribed medications, but the process should be completely transparent, including informing people of potential side effects and withdrawal problems. No one should ever be told they are being prescribed drugs to treat a genetically caused schizophrenia brain disease—not the "patient," not the family, not anyone.

Genetic determinists worry about reproduction patterns and what they see as the societal burden of mental disorders, whereas many environmentalists focus on what they see as the mental burden of societal disorders. Currently, most people interested in or involved in the "genetics of schizophrenia" topic fall somewhere in between the genetic determinist and environmentalist positions, and most people believe that a genetic predisposition of some type is necessary. There is a wide range of opinion related to causes, prevention, and interventions ("treatments"). While recognizing that most people currently fall into this "somewhere in between" position, I will now focus on selected authors and groups who have opposed the disease model.

Thomas Szasz

Critical psychiatrist Thomas Szasz (1920–2012), the author of *The Myth of Mental Illness*, pointed out in 1976 that instead of focusing on what Kraepelin and Bleuler *believed* about biological causes, contemporary commentators should instead focus on these investigators' "utter inability to support their beliefs with a shred of relevant *evidence*."[5] What Kraepelin and Bleuler helped to accomplish, in Szasz's view, was to "subtly ... redefine the criterion of disease, from histopathology [pathology of tissues] to psychopathology–that is, from abnormal bodily structure to abnormal personal behavior."[6] This lies at the core of modern psychiatric medical model approaches, where dysfunctional or socially disapproved personal behaviors are transformed into discrete diseases or disorders, largely downplaying psychological and social contexts in the process.

Szasz repeatedly pointed out that when a "mental disorder" is shown to be caused by a brain disease, it leaves the realm of psychiatry and becomes the concern of other branches of medicine, such as neurology. In cases where brain pathology is proven—and not just claimed—medical science recognizes that the person has a brain disease, not a mental disorder.[7] "Mental illness does not exist not because no one has yet found such a disease," Szasz wrote, "but because *no one can find such a disease*: the only kind of disease medical researchers can find is literal, bodily disease."[8] If "schizophrenia is a brain disease," Szasz once asked, "why do the scientists at the [U.S.] National Institute of *Mental Health*, rather than those at the National Institute of *Neurological Diseases*, tell us that?"[9]

David Hill

In his 1983 work *The Politics of Schizophrenia: Psychiatric Oppression in the United States*, David Hill saw reductionist approaches as serving a social control aspect of psychiatry, which in his view involved four components. The first is the "establishment of certain norms by either the majority or the powerful, and the breaking of those norms by a relatively powerless minority." The second aspect of social control is "an exaggeration of the difference between the 'in-group' and the 'out group'…by the application of the medical dichotomy 'sick-healthy' to behaviors, followed by ignoring the context of those behaviors, thereby rendering them even more bizarre." The third control aspect "is presented as benevolent concern; accomplished by the portrayal of those exhibiting the strange behaviors as not being responsible for them; this in turn being explained by some supposed physiological or hereditary etiology or by some disorder of volition or will." These three aspects lead to the fourth component, "the implementation of sanctions called, in this particular case, 'psychiatric treatment.'"[10]

John Read

Psychologist John Read and colleagues described the position of some authors, who like Hill have argued that one role of modern psychiatry "is to sweep up the social casualties of Western industrialized societies by re-defining their difficulties as individual, biologically-based 'illnesses' … and applying 'treatments' that silence and disable people even further."[11] Read saw "schizophrenia" as a "scientifically meaningless and socially devastating label."[12]

Read and colleagues' "Traumagenic Neurodevelopmental" (TN) model of psychosis highlights "processes by which childhood adversities may lead to symptoms of psychosis later in life," and "proposes that the heightened sensitivity to stress consistently found in people diagnosed with psychotic disorders including schizophrenia originates, for many patients, in neurodevelomental changes to the brain caused by trauma in the early years."[13]

The Power Threat Meaning Framework *(PTMF)*

In contrast to mainstream views, non-medical approaches stress the role of the family and the larger culture and society, including racial and other types of oppression, in causing psychosis. The idea of schizophrenia as a medical condition is rejected. Another example of this approach is the *Power Threat Meaning Framework* (PTMF), developed by Lucy Johnstone, Mary Boyle, and others.[14] In a 2020 introductory book, the authors described the Framework's "overall message" as follows:

> All forms of adversity and distress are more common in social contexts of inequality and other forms of deprivation, discrimination, marginalisation and injustice. This evidence does not support the individualisation of distress, either medically or psychologically. Instead, it implies the need for action, primarily through social policy, at the earliest possible point, before the destructive and self-perpetuating cycles are set in motion.[15]

Psychiatry sees a person exhibiting psychotic behavior, and in step with the medical model asks: "What is *wrong* with you?" The PTMF asks, as do most psychotherapists, "What *happened* to you?" It also offers a way of integrating the social, psychological and biological, but very differently from either the disease or the biopsychosocial models. Given the lack of evidence, terms such as "brain disease," "genetic predisposition," "genes," "twin and adoption studies," and "heritability" should not be found in the answer to either of the above questions.

Implications for Clinical Practice and Prevention

Primary Prevention

Primary prevention "aims to prevent disease or injury before it occurs. This is done by preventing exposures to hazards that cause disease or injury, altering unhealthy or unsafe behaviors that can lead to disease or injury, and increasing resistance to disease or injury should exposure occur."[16]

For example, lung cancer primary prevention programs attempt to convince people through public service campaigns that smoking tobacco can cause lung cancer, with the goal being to convince people to not smoke tobacco as a way of preventing lung cancer. Schizophrenia and other psychiatric conditions are not diseases, but the basic idea applies.

The approach to schizophrenia and psychosis primary prevention depends, of course, on one's beliefs about the causes. Supporters of biological and genetic theories focus on human reproduction patterns and psychiatric genetic counseling programs, and tertiary prevention methods such a prescribing and improving neuroleptic medication. Supporters of environmental theories reject the disease model and focus on improving people's environments, and mitigating, reducing, or eliminating the environmental factors I discussed in Chapter 1. We saw that these include experiencing emotional abuse, incest, neglect, parental loss, physical abuse, sexual abuse, poverty, racism, migratory stress, and urbanicity. In addition, focus could be placed on changing experiences related to the mother's health, nutrition, and stress during pregnancy; being the product of an unwanted pregnancy; early loss of parents via death or abandonment; separation of parents; witnessing interparental violence; dysfunctional parenting (often intergenerational); war trauma; rape or physical assaults as an adult; and racial and other forms of discrimination and oppression.

A well-known environmentalist in his field, psychologist George Albee (1921–2006) advocated primary prevention approaches, with an unavoidable political component. Because "many mental disorders are socially acquired maladjustments, learned patterns of undesirable behavior that result from a pathological social environment," wrote Albee, "logically, prevention programs should include efforts at achieving social equality for all...but such efforts threaten the status quo and so are not part of the prevention agenda."[17] Clearly, "achieving social equality for all" is an intervention with positive implications for people's overall psychological well-being.

Psychiatrist Joanna Moncrieff wrote that because

> we know that poverty, unemployment, insecure attachments, familial disruption, low self-esteem, abuse etc. play a role [in causing psychosis] we would be better concentrating on how to eliminate these from our society if we really want to reduce the impact of mental disorder, rather than pouring more money into the bottomless pit of genetic research.[18]

This conclusion is consistent with a recognition that, for the foreseeable future, people diagnosed with schizophrenia and psychosis will continue to be prescribed and use neuroleptic ("anti-psychotic") medications. However, the fact that in some cases these drugs help people function better in their daily lives supplies no evidence that the drugs are treating a disease.

Prevention efforts must address racism, sexism, poverty, the mistreatment of sexual minorities, and other forms of oppression. Yet governments, corporations, drug companies, and the psychiatric establishments promote approaches that focus on genes and brains in the process of *depoliticizing* human suffering. As James Davies wrote in *Sedated: How Modern Capitalism Created Our Mental Health Crisis*, these groups "conceptualise human suffering in ways that protect the current economy from criticism," by framing "suffering as being rooted in individual rather than social causes...."[19]

The powers that be promote bad science to help turn our attention away from harmful social conditions, political policy decisions, bloated military budgets, and the concentration of wealth in the hands of a few. Even before the COVID-19 pandemic, the world's 2,153 billionaires had accumulated more wealth than held by the poorest 60 percent of the planet's population.[20] Redistributing some of that wealth would do wonders for people's mental health.

Alternative Intervention Methods and Approaches

I now briefly describe some interventions and approaches developed as alternatives to medical models of schizophrenia and psychosis. It is beyond the scope of this chapter to review outcome research based on these interventions and approaches.

Soteria House

The *Soteria* program was established by psychiatrist Loren Mosher (1933–2004) as an alternative to medical-model approaches for first-episode psychosis. Mosher was the head of the Center for Studies of Schizophrenia in the 1970s, a department of the U.S. National Institute for Mental Health (NIMH). He was the founder and first Editor-in-chief of *Schizophrenia Bulletin*. Soteria House opened its doors in 1971. The first building was a vintage 12-room house located in a residential neighborhood in the San Jose area of California. A similar facility was opened in another part of the San Francisco Bay Area three years later. Soteria's core principles were developed by Mosher and Luc Ciompi over a 30-year period, and included:

> (1) the provision of a small, community-based therapeutic milieu (akin to a living community); (2) a significant proportion of lay person staff; (3) the preservation of personal power, social networks, and communal responsibilities; (4) a "phenomenological" relational style which aims to give meaning to a person's subjective experience of psychosis by developing an understanding of it by "being with" and "doing with" the clients; and (5) no or low-dose antipsychotic medication, with all psychotropic medications being taken by choice and without coercion.[21]

Soteria was loosely based on R. D. Laing's earlier Kingsley Hall program in London. As Mosher and his colleague John Bola described it, the "essential characteristics of Soteria included a small staff, home-like atmosphere, peer/fraternal relationship orientation to minimize authority, minimal hierarchy, open social system allowing departure and return if needed, post-discharge continuity of relationships encouraged, no formal 'therapy.'"[22]

The Soteria model presented a challenge to the psychiatric establishment and the pharmaceutical industry, which Mosher summarized in three refreshing principles: "One, Soteria called into question the medical model: it said, whatever schizophrenia is, we don't believe it's a medical illness. Two, if schizophrenia isn't a medical problem, it doesn't need to be treated in hospital. ...And three – no neuroleptics."[23]

The U.S. Soteria program shut down in 1983 due to a lack of funding, amid American psychiatry's turn to a much greater emphasis on biological explanations and treatments. The NIMH cut off all funding for Soteria, and Mosher was pushed out of his job there. The clear message, as Robert Whitaker wrote in words that echo the experience of Theodore Lidz's adoption study critiques, was that "those who did not get behind the biomedical model would not have much of a future."[24] In 1984 a Soteria replication was established by Ciompi in Switzerland. Soteria-like programs have been established in other countries.[25]

Mosher later resigned from the American Psychiatric Association. The following passages are found in his letter of resignation, dated December 4, 1998:

> This is not a group for me. At this point in history, in my view, psychiatry has been almost completely bought out by the drug companies. The APA could not continue without the pharmaceutical company support of meetings, symposia, workshops, journal advertising, grand rounds luncheons, unrestricted educational grants etc. etc. Psychiatrists have become the minions of drug company promotions. APA, of course, maintains that its independence and autonomy are not compromised in this enmeshed situation.

> Biologically based brain diseases are convenient for families and practitioners alike. It is no fault insurance against personal responsibility. We are just helplessly caught up in a swirl of brain pathology for which no one, except DNA, is responsible. Now, to begin with, anything that has an anatomically defined specific brain pathology becomes the province of neurology (syphilis is an excellent example). So, to be consistent with this "brain disease" view all the major psychiatric disorders would become the territory of our neurologic colleagues. ...The fact that there is no evidence confirming the brain disease attribution is, at this point, irrelevant. What we are dealing with here is fashion, politics and money. This level of intellectual/scientific dishonesty is just too egregious for me to continue to support by my membership.[26]

The Hearing Voices Movement (HVM)

The experience of hearing voices is more common than most people think.[27] Psychiatry calls these "auditory hallucinations," and sees them as a symptom of a context-free "schizophrenia disease" in need of medication. The *Hearing Voices Movement* (HVM), which began in The Netherlands in the 1980s, takes the approach that hearing voices does not necessarily mean that people who hear them are experiencing psychosis. The HVM sees voice hearing not as a sign of mental illness, but as "significant, decipherable, and intimately connected to a person's life story."[28]

A 2017 article described the five HVM "core principles":

> (1) hearing voices is not in itself indicative of pathology or mental illness, but rather a real and meaningful experience; (2) many individuals who hear voices do not have symptoms that would lead to a diagnosis of mental illness, nor have they needed to seek psychiatric services; (3) hearing voices is most often related to adverse life experiences, commonly trauma or abuse; (4) those individuals who are distressed by their voices can come to an understanding of the voices that lessens their distress (i.e., the voices become more manageable, if not helpful at times), and; (5) the voice hearer's ability to cope is often strengthened by confronting the negative experiences in his or her past that initially led to the development of the voices.[29]

Hearing Voices Network peer-support groups operate in many countries, and offer support and guidance while rejecting medical and pathologizing approaches to voice hearing.

Open Dialogue

The *Open Dialogue* approach to first-episode psychosis was developed in Finland in the 1980s. The method is described below:

> Dedicated to giving immediate help in a crisis, the basic format of the Open Dialogue is the treatment meeting, which occurs within twenty-four hours of the initial contact. It is organized by a mobile crisis team composed of outpatient and inpatient staff and takes place, if possible, at the family home. It brings together the person in acute distress with the team and all other important persons (i.e., relatives, friends, and other professionals) connected to the situation. The meeting takes place physically in an open forum as well, with everyone sitting in the same room, in a circle.[30]

Open Dialogue was developed as an alternative to the standard practice of distressed people going to or being taken to a psychiatric emergency facility and being treated there as if they had a medical condition.

Cognitive Behavioral Therapy for Psychosis (CBTp)

In the 1960s Aaron Beck (1921–2021) developed Cognitive Therapy, based on the idea that dysfunctional thinking leads to negative feelings and unwanted behavior. This led to the development of Cognitive Behavioral Therapy for Psychosis (CBTp). A goal of CBTp is to "focus on generating less distressing explanations for psychotic experiences, rather than attempting to eliminate these experiences." CBTp practitioners recognize that "psychotic experiences may well serve a function for the person."[31] As Read and colleagues described it,

> CBT for psychosis (CBTp) is a collaborative and problem-orientated approach, working toward goals identified by the patient.[23] Given the prevalence of adversity and childhood/adult trauma, it is unsurprising that a significant proportion of the work involves trauma-focused interventions. There is a recognition that CBTp should address traumatic experiences and should acknowledge and validate the influence such experiences have on current mental health.[32]

Although CBTp is a non-medical approach, it is sometimes incorporated into standard psychiatric medication + CBT treatment strategies. This mainstream perspective sees CBTp as a component of the "stress vulnerability" (diathesis-stress) model, where we have seen that the "vulnerability" aspect refers to an assumed genetic predisposition.[33] In 2002, Boyle referred to this process as the "assimilation and neutralisation" of CBTp by medical model practitioners.[34]

* * *

Having surveyed schizophrenia genetic research in the previous chapters, and some alternative perspectives in this chapter, I now close with some final comments.

A World without Schizophrenia Genes

Genes that play a role in causing schizophrenia exist in the public and scientific imagination but are unlikely to exist in reality. In my first "genetics of schizophrenia" article, which was published in 1999, I concluded, "Based on the weight of the evidence, it is predicted here that a gene for schizophrenia will not be found, because it does not exist."[35] I continue to predict that genes that play a direct role in causing schizophrenia or psychosis will never be found, because there is no reason to believe that such genes exist.

In response to 1970s-era critics of psychiatry and the schizophrenia concept such as Szasz, Laing, and Peter Breggin, in 1974 Seymour Kety pointed specifically to his adoption study's biological paternal half-sibling comparison as providing "compelling evidence" that schizophrenia exists, and that genes play a major role. "If schizophrenia is a myth," wrote Kety, with Szasz clearly in mind, "it is a myth with a strong genetic component!"[36] I showed in Chapter 6 that Kety openly manipulated his biological paternal half-sibling comparison to arrive at that conclusion, apparently seeing nothing wrong with the practice of temporarily removing a "schizophrenia spectrum" diagnosis to achieve statistically significant results. Many years later, Kety's "myth with a strong genetic component" statement reads like an exemplar of bad science. Based on the analysis I presented in previous chapters, we can now adjust Kety's unapologetically p-hacked conclusion to read as follows—*If schizophrenia is a genetic disorder, it is a genetic disorder with a strong mythical component!*

The story is not so much about genes as it is about the people who do schizophrenia genetic research, and the people who write about this research. Genes didn't create a "disease" for which different people can display completely different behaviors ("symptoms"). Irrelevant genes don't call themselves candidate genes. Genes don't say that chance or spurious associations with "schizophrenia" suggest gene discovery. Genes didn't insert the phrase "trait relevant" into the definition of the twin method's equal environment assumption to keep behavioral twin research alive, and genes don't assume that MZ and DZ twin environments are "equal" when everyone knows they aren't equal. Genes didn't transform 15 percent MZ schizophrenia concordance into a 79 percent heritability estimate. Genes didn't continue to look for more adoptees and relatives when an adoption study found no genetic influences. No gene ever changed adoption study comparisons after seeing that the planned comparison led to undesired conclusions, and no gene temporarily removed a schizophrenia spectrum disorder category from a key adoption study comparison to achieve statistically significant results. Genes don't count people judged only as being a "pervert" as having a schizophrenia spectrum disorder. Genes don't utilize QRPs or have financial conflicts of interest, and genes don't write textbooks and other key publications overlooking QRPs and financial conflicts of interest. Genes don't say that environmental factors are "mysterious," nor do they minimize or deny the psychologically harmful impact of severe and prolonged childhood sexual and other types of abuse. No gene ever cited "fleets" of schizophrenia twin studies that don't exist, and genes don't write psychiatry textbooks citing nonexistent studies.

These are all things that *people* have done, and if people hadn't done these things, few people would be looking for or talking about "schizophrenia genes."

I mentioned at the end of Chapter 1 sociologist Howard Taylor's 1980 description of "The IQ Game." To review, Taylor was describing IQ-genetic researchers' "use of assumptions that are implausible as well as arbitrary to arrive at some numerical value for the genetic heritability of human IQ scores on the grounds that no heritability calculations could be made without benefit of such assumptions."[37] Modifying Taylor's description to fit schizophrenia genetic research and claims, in this book I have described the use of false or questionable assumptions, p-hacking, HARKing, and other questionable research practices, and the promotion of spurious or non-causative "gene association" claims to produce schizophrenia heritability estimates and gene discovery claims, because no such estimates or claims could be made without engaging in such practices. *This is the schizophrenia game.* It has been played for over a century, and it's time to stop. A world without schizophrenia genes will do just fine.

Notes

1 Ioannidis, J. (2005), Why Most Published Research Findings are False, *PLoS Medicine, 2,* 696–701, p. 700. https://doi.org/10.1371/journal.pmed.0020124
2 Bentall, R. P. (2009), *Doctoring the Mind: Is Our Current Treatment of Mental Illness Really Any Good?*, New York: New York University Press, p. 145.
3 Rogers, A. (2017, May 11th), Star Neuroscientist Tom Insel Leaves the Google-Spawned Verily for … a Startup?, *Wired.* https://www.wired.com/2017/05/star-neuroscientist-tom-insel-leaves-google-spawned-verily-startup/
4 Scull, A. (2022), *Desperate Remedies: Psychiatry's Turbulent Quest to Cure Mental Illness,* Cambridge, MA: Belknap Press, p. 380.
5 Szasz, T. S. (1961), *The Myth of Mental Illness: Foundations of a Theory of Personal Conduct,* New York: Hoeber-Harper.
6 Szasz, T. S. (1976), *Schizophrenia: The Sacred Symbol of Psychiatry,* New York: Basic Books, p. 12.
7 Szasz, T. S. (1997), *Insanity: The Idea and its Consequences,* Syracuse, NY: Syracuse University Press (originally published in 1987).
8 Szasz, T. S. (2004), Reply to Bentall, in J. Schaler (Ed.), *Szasz Under Fire: The Psychiatric Abolitionist Faces His Critics* (pp. 321–353), Chicago: Open Court, p. 322.
9 Szasz, 1997, p. 50.
10 Hill, D. (1983), *The Politics of Schizophrenia: Psychiatric Oppression in the United States,* Lanham, MD: University Press of America, p. 104.
11 Read, J., Johnstone, L., & Taitimu, M. (2013), Psychosis, Poverty and Ethnicity, in J. Read & J. Dillon (Eds.), *Models of Madness: Psychological, Social and Biological Approaches to Psychosis* (2nd ed., pp. 191–209), London: Routledge, p. 205.
12 Read, J. (2013), The Invention of Schizophrenia, in J. Read & J. Dillon (Eds.), *Models of Madness: Psychological, Social and Biological Approaches to Psychosis* (2nd ed., pp. 20–33), London: Routledge, p. 32.
13 Read et al. (2014), The Traumagenic Neurodevelopmental Model of Psychosis Revisited, *Neuropsychiatry, 4,* 65–79, p. 66. https://doi.org/10.2217/NPY.13.89
14 For Power Threat Meaning Framework (PTMF) documents, see https://www.bps.org.uk/power-threat-meaning-framework
15 Boyle, M., & Johnstone, L. (2020), *A Straight Talking Introduction to the Power Threat Meaning Framework: An Alternative to Psychiatric Diagnosis,* Monmouth, UK: PCCS Books, p. 105.
16 Institute for Work & Health (online publication), Primary, Secondary, and Tertiary Prevention. https://www.iwh.on.ca/what-researchers-mean-by/primary-secondary-and-tertiary-prevention#:~:text=Primary%20prevention%20aims%20to%20prevent,or%20injury%20should%20exposure%20occur.
17 Albee, G. W. (1996), Revolutions and Counterrevolutions in Prevention, *American Psychologist, 51,* 1130–1133, pp. 1130, 1132. https://doi.org/10.1037//0003-066x.51.11.1130
18 Moncrieff, J. (2014, September 1), A Critique of Genetic Research on Schizophrenia – Expensive Castles in the Air, [Web log post]. https://joannamoncrieff.com/2014/09/01/a-critique-of-genetic-research-on-schizophrenia-expensive-castles-in-the-air/
19 Davies, J. (2021), *Sedated: How Modern Capitalism Created Our Mental Health Crisis,* London: Atlantic Books, p. 34.
20 Oxfam International (2020, January 20th), World's Billionaires Have More Wealth Than 4.6 Billion People. https://www.oxfam.org/en/press-releases/worlds-billionaires-have-more-wealth-46-billion-people

21 Calton et al. (2008), A Systematic Review of the Soteria Paradigm for the Treatment of People Diagnosed with Schizophrenia, *Schizophrenia Bulletin, 34*, 181–192, p. 181. https://doi.org/10.1093/schbul/sbm047

22 Mosher, L. R. (2004), Non-hospital, Non-drug Intervention with First-episode Psychosis, in J. Read, L. Mosher, & R. Bentall (Eds.), *Models of Madness: Psychological, Social and Biological Approaches to Schizophrenia* (pp. 349–364), Andover, UK: Taylor & Francis, p. 365.

23 Mosher, L. R. (2004, April, interview), Lone Voice, *Mental Health Today*, 18.

24 Whitaker, R. (2010), *Anatomy of an Epidemic: Magic Bullets, Psychiatric Drugs, and the Astonishing Rise of Mental Illness in America*. New York: Crown, p. 272.

25 Bergner, D. (2022, May 17ᵗʰ), Doctors Gave Her Antipsychotics. She Decided to Live with Her Voices, *New York Times*. https://www.nytimes.com/2022/05/17/magazine/antipsychotic-medications-mental-health.html

26 http://www.narpa.org/reference/mosher

27 Boyle, M. (2002), *Schizophrenia: A Scientific Delusion?* (2nd ed.), Hove, UK: Routledge, Chapter 8.

28 Dillon et al. (2013), The Work of Experienced-Based Experts, in J. Read & J. Dillon (Eds.), *Models of Madness: Psychological, Social and Biological Approaches to Psychosis* (2nd ed., pp. 305–318), London: Routledge, p. 313.

29 Styron, T., Utter, L., & Davidson, L. (2017), The Hearing Voices Network: Initial Lessons and Future Directions for Mental Health Professionals and Systems of Care, *Psychiatric Quarterly, 88*, 769–785, pp. 773–774. https://doi.org/10.1007/s11126-017-9491-1

30 Seikkula, J., & Olson, M. E. (2003), The Open Dialogue Approach to Acute Psychosis: Its Poetics and Micropolitics, *Family Process, 42*, 403–418, p. 406. https://doi.org/10.1111/j.1545-5300.2003.00403.x

31 Morrison, A. (2013), Cognitive Therapy for People Experiencing Psychosis, in J. Read & J. Dillon (Eds.), *Models of Madness: Psychological, Social and Biological Approaches to Psychosis* (2nd ed., pp. 319–335), London: Routledge, p. 320.

32 Read et al. (2020), Traumas, Adversities, and Psychosis: Investigating Practical Implications, *Psychiatric Times, 37*. https://www.psychiatrictimes.com/view/traumas-adversities-and-psychosis-investigating-practical-implications

33 For example, see Landa, Y. (2017), Cognitive Behavioral Therapy for Psychosis (CBTp): An Introductory Manual for Clinicians. https://www.mirecc.va.gov/visn2/docs/CBTp_Manual_VA_Yulia_Landa_2017.pdf

34 Boyle, 2002, p. 312.

35 Joseph, J. (1999), The Genetic Theory of Schizophrenia: A Critical Overview, *Ethical Human Sciences and Services, 1*, 119–145, p. 137.

36 Kety, S. S. (1974), From Rationalization to Reason, *American Journal of Psychiatry, 131*, 957–963, p. 961. https://doi.org/10.1176/ajp.131.9.957,

37 Taylor, H. F. (1980), *The IQ Game: A Methodological Inquiry into the Heredity-Environment Controversy*, New Brunswick, NJ: Rutgers University Press, p. 7.

Index

Page numbers in **bold** indicate a table on the corresponding page